Jogging

How to Start Running for Weight Loss

(A Collection of Comic Strips Loosely Themed on Running)

Elbert Carrion

Published By **Elena Holly**

Elbert Carrion

Jogging: How to Start Running for Weight Loss (A Collection of Comic Strips Loosely Themed on Running)

ISBN 978-1-7752436-7-0

No part of this guidebook shall be reproduced in any form without permission in writing from the publisher except in the case of brief quotations embodied in critical articles or reviews.

Legal & Disclaimer

The information contained in this book is not designed to replace or take the place of any form of medicine or professional medical advice. The information in this book has been provided for educational & entertainment purposes only.

The information contained in this book has been compiled from sources deemed reliable, and it is accurate to the best of the Author's knowledge; however, the Author cannot guarantee its accuracy and validity and cannot be held liable for any errors or omissions. Changes are periodically made to this book. You must consult your doctor or get professional medical advice before using any of the suggested remedies, techniques, or information in this book.

Table Of Contents

Chapter 1: Metabolism And How It Works

A few people work out and reduce calories consumed in search for weight loss, and then end up being frustrated. One of the reasons that most of us are here and remain there is mainly due to their lower metabolism. It is good to know you are able to control the metabolism rate of your body with workouts that work your body, and boost your speed of metabolism.

Metabolism is a chemical procedure by which the body's body eliminates unwanted fat that is stored in our bodies, giving us the energy needed to complete certain essential activities. The rate at which this happens, is dependent on the exercises is performed in the gym as well as the exercises we perform in the outside world without knowing about it.

The base metabolic rate represents the energy level the body needs for the tasks described above.

Fats that are burnt provide us with the ability to perform the tasks is normal for us, such as be active, thinking and exercise. The energy you get from burning fats for all sorts of tasks. With an increased activity level, you require an increase in energy. This means greater fat burning.

What Determines the Rate of Metabolism?

Certain factors determine your metabolism's basal rate, which means you don't need to be concerned if it isn't high enough since you can effortlessly increase it. Your body's weight the gender of your body, your age, as well as genetics are just a few of the elements that determine how high or low your metabolism is likely to be.

* Body Size

They require less energy to burn as compared to their equivalents (muscle,) this means that individuals with plenty of muscle will be more active that those who have lots of fats.

* Age

When a person's body gets older, it is prone to shed muscle mass and increase fat, which is the reason metabolism rates tend to drop when you get older.

* Gender

Men are more likely to have bigger muscles as well as less body fat, and have larger bones than women. That is why men are more active and also have higher calories consumed.

* Genes

It is also believed that they contribute to the human's metabolism, but this isn't really understood and demonstrated about how this happens.

Many people with obesity often blame their rate of metabolism of why they've plenty of fat. However, in large body mass metabolic rate is high enough to supply the energy requirements for their bodies.

If you fall into this class, the most important reason your weight loss is not happening by boosting your metabolism is likely to be because you're eating more calories than ones your body is burning. This results in the accumulation of fat in your body to be used later. usage. Cut down on your consumption and start training and you'll shortly be on the path to that beach figure you're looking for.

Certain ailments and illnesses which can slow down the metabolic rate of your body. A few of them are Cushing's and hypothyroidism. If you suspect that your metabolism may be low because of a illness, it is recommended to see your physician for an appropriate assessment and treatment.

Faster Metabolism

The speed that you use up your fats will depend on the rate of your metabolism. When you boost your metabolic rate, you'll are losing more fats. It is possible to boost the speed of your metabolism, to the point that your body will be burning off fats all day long, which implies that you'll get rid of the extra weight quickly and be into shape.

An exercise program that is properly executed and a balanced diet will boost the body's metabolism by around 5 to 6 hundreds of calories daily. Your body will always burn calories. All you have to do to drop pounds as quickly according to your desires is get better at adjusting your body's metabolism by using the right type of workout.

The pace of our metabolism will depend depending on gender an individual as well as their genetic composition. The exercises women perform won't necessarily suit men and vice versa, so be sure that you are aware of the regimen of exercises that be beneficial for you.

Tips For Speeding Up Your Metabolism

Less but Frequent Exercise

It's been proved by athletes and scientists that when you do a few ten minute exercise sessions, you can shed more pounds than you would if you do a 30 minutes of exercise. Smaller workouts help boost your metabolism over longer durations of time and result in the burning of additional fats.

The After Burn

Afterburn is the capacity for the body to continue burning off fats even after the training. The harder your exercise will be, the more calories you burn, and will continue to burn them even after leaving the fitness center.

There are a variety of high-intensity interval exercises for increased metabolism-burning rate. The benefit of such workouts is that they'll keep your body burning calories for 12 to forty-eight hours following the exercise. It means that you'll lose more fat and shed more weight quicker and with less risk.

They are beneficial and must be performed regularly. It is possible to incorporate moderately intense workouts in between so that you can get rid of fats more effective.

Drinking Lots of Water

It is suggested to drink at least 1 liter of water each daily. It prevents the bloating that can occur and improves the rate of metabolism. Additionally, it flushes excess water from your body. A glass of chilled water is the most effective option as it causes your metabolic rate increasing by your body to heat it up.

The research shows that metabolism inside your body increases to thirty percent over the following ten minutes after drinking cold water.

Foods that contain greater protein and fiber.

If your body is processing food items that contain high levels of protein and fiber in general, it increases the metabolic rate to ensure that it can handle it easily. Take in foods with a higher amount of complex carbohydrates and more than 30 percent protein at each meal, and your metabolism will increase dramatically.

Morning Workouts

Exercise early in the morning is the most effective thing you can take if you're looking to shed some weight. This also aids to kick-start your metabolism while keeping it up throughout the day. Therefore, if you're trying to shed some weight in a brief amount of time, consider getting up early in the morning before working by doing a vigorous workout to get beneficial after-burn benefits for the rest of the day.

Exercise in the evening is good, but they're not ideal as the metabolism rate is likely to slow when you fall asleep. Make sure you complete your workouts early in the morning and you'll be in the process of achieving the body you want.

Skipping Breakfast

Breakfast is considered to be the most crucial food of the day since it will give you the necessary energy to get through the day. If you don't eat breakfast, your body will be required to search for a fuel source and is able to burn calories to provide your energy requirements throughout the day.

The human growth hormone (HGM)

It is a hormone which helps you build muscle mass and keep them in shape. This procedure requires energy, and a higher level of metabolism that is taking place in the body. If you're able to raise the levels of HGM present in your body you'll not just lose weight but also gain nice looking muscles.

Work on Gaining Muscle

For every pound of muscle that you have in your body, can burn anywhere between six and 12 pounds of calories per day. As you build up your muscles and the greater number of calories you can burn because all of the muscles need your body to work harder to recover them from any workout you did. Muscles boost the metabolism of your body and it will be beneficial to increase your muscle mass.

Green Tea

A research study in the US found that people who consumed green tea for 3 months lost nearly two times more weight than who didn't consume the green tea. Green tea will assist you to reduce between thirty-five and forty-three more calories per daily. Green tea is also beneficial to overall health. So change to green tea if you're not currently on green tea.

Be Active

That is to say that you should must always be active and don't allow your body to stay at a permanent state. Being active in your body makes it capable of burning calories in a continuous manner If you're used of taking the bus to work or if you live close to your workplace You can walk to and from work, or walk home after your job.

Spices

The results of studies have proven that the use of spices increase your metabolism by around twenty percent within 30 minutes after you consume these. Incorporate a couple of milligrams of cayenne pepper, or anything similar to spicy mustard into your meals and you'll soon be on the journey to having a higher metabolic rate for a while. The heat of the spices will increase the speed of metabolism, which results in greater fat burning within the body.

Thyroid Function

The thyroid gland is responsible in regulating the metabolism of your body.

The consumption of fish and nuts that are rich in vitamins E, Iodine, Copper, Selenium and Zinc will boost the function of your thyroid. This will increase the speed of metabolism.

Insufficient nutrients immediately slow the metabolism of your body. And can lead to formation of hypothyroidism.

Caffeine Consumption

Moderate consumption (which amounts to between 50 and 300mg or 2 cups) of caffeine can raise the metabolic rate of your body. The caffeine produces adrenaline, which can help increase the metabolism of your body. This will aid to burn more fats when you exercise.

It's good to be aware that every workout you perform have a degree of an afterburn result. The effect that follows burn from intense exercises is the sole one that keeps the rate of metabolism that burns calories up and maintains them over a prolonged amount of duration.

Training sessions of around ten minutes in intervals throughout the day can be better at achieving the post-burn effect which keeps your body burning off fats throughout the day long, as opposed to a forty-minute exercise.

Chapter 2: Nutrition Tips For Pre And Post Workout

In order to shed weight, you need an entire plan that allows the user to eliminate the extra fat and keep your muscles. The issue with insane diets or pursuing an exercise program that restricts calories is that you'll reduce the metabolic rate at which you basalize which will result in that your muscles are being sucked up for energy production that your body can use.

These crash diets can cause a reduction in muscle mass your body. In turn, your metabolism will slow down, which can lead to your body increasing fats after you've finished the program. The best advice I can give you is to avoid these crazy plans and aim to eliminate those fats in a sustainable and healthier method.

Post-Workout Nutrition Tips

Proteins are among the most important and essential kinds of foods for losing weight. One of the most important factors in successful weight loss does not mean exercising for hours on end or going to the gym and using weights. It can depend on the food you eat prior to and following your exercise. A healthy diet is the simplest method to ensure that you shed the fats don't need while also gaining muscle mass or preserve your existing ones.

The combination of sprinting exercises along with a balanced protein diet comes from the belief that it is necessary to consume large quantities of protein to enhance muscles' protein synthesis. If they are combined, they create an effect that is synergistic and it's recommended to consume protein after your exercise. It is due to the fact that muscles are activated through strong contractions in the muscles that you already possess.

The best dosage of protein will be between twenty-five grams. The ten grams originate from amino acids. Forty percent will be from leucine. It is an amino acid that is a branched chain.

Leucine amino acids enhance protein synthesis for all of a period of time following a workout. This makes milk proteins more beneficial over those from other foods like soy. A large intake of protein in the elderly are better for their health, though this is still to be confirmed scientifically.

The protein content of Whey is definitely than other types due to their speedy digesting patterns as well as their fact that they contain plenty of leucine. Hypertrophy is a problem that affects both men and women as well as for seniors.

It is possible that the proteins may help the development of muscles when in a specific physiological situation or in individuals, but this is not a confirmed theory also.

Researchers have developed suggestions on the best way to consume the protein you consume to get the most benefit you can reap from them. Check out the suggestions below suggestions and test it out and you can be beneficial to you in conjunction with the training program for sprints.

I. The best amount of protein grams/kg of weight should range between 0.25 or 0.3. These should be quality proteins included in each meal you eat.

II. The main predictor for the protein synthesis reaction after meals is the level of leucine present of the meal. Be sure to take huge amounts of it in every meal.

III. Protein synthesis during the night can be accomplished by ensuring that you consume a protein prior to going to go to bed.

IV. To get the most effective food source after a exercise, ensure that you eat some protein-rich whey.

V. A. Consumption of one-sixth of a gram of protein per kilogram your body weight can accelerate the reduction of fat.

Some Foods for Fat Loss and Body Composition

The food items we'll discuss here will be beneficial in achieving effective fat loss, and helping you achieve the ideal body you could ever have. If you incorporate them into every meal, they'll prove to be extremely beneficial for the person eating them, since they are essentially plenty of protein, nutritious carbs, and fats that can aid in gaining weight and feel energetic throughout the day.

The items that are in question comprise however are not restricted to:

Cold Water Fish

They include fish, such as whitefish and salmon, as well as sardines, mackerel, and anchovies. They're high in omega-3 fats, which can help in reducing inflammation as well as increasing the insulin sensitivity. An increase in insulin sensitivity will help your body to store carbs that you consume in the form of glycogen in your muscles, not in the forms of fats.

A decrease in inflammation can lead to a more balanced metabolism hormone balance and results in you feeling fuller and an increased metabolism. It is also likely you are more satisfied with food and feel more satisfied when you consume food.

This has been proven by several studies conducted that demonstrated that daily consumption of at least 4 grams of omega-3 over 1 1/2 months resulted in an increase in lean mass and a reduction in fats within the body.

Nuts

The consumption of nuts like almonds and walnuts that are rich in antioxidants, fiber, health oils and protein, is an effective way to shed undesirable fats. By incorporating some of these nuts can help you to improve your body's composition dramatically. They not only increase metabolism but enhance the sense of fullness and decrease appetite.

Raw walnuts are eaten and with the skin on making them the healthiest of nuts as have a high amount of antioxidants. They also contain high levels of levels of protein as well as vitamin E and fiber levels, which makes them ideal for waste removal from your body.

At least one amount of nuts per day can boost the loss of fat and make you feel satisfied.

Berries

This includes berries like blueberries as well as strawberries, raspberries, and blueberries; aside from their delicious taste, they're great at shedding pounds as they're loaded with antioxidants and fiber. They can also improve the quantity of insulin your body makes due to high carbohydrate diets. Ellagitannins are an antioxidant that is that is found in the raspberries. It helps people be less hungry due to the improvement of the brain's response to leptin.

It is important to ensure that you at the very least, have two portions of berries throughout the day. You could incorporate other fruits like the pomegranate, mango and tart cherries for an array of flavors. Nobody wants to consume the same meal cooked the same manner.

Avocados

The avocado fruit has a powerful antioxidant, and is a powerful antioxidant. It is also an excellent fruit for reducing obesity. The avocado has around 2500 calories and ten milligrams of fiber 4 grams of protein, 20 important nutrients, and fifteen pounds of monounsaturated fats.

Whey Protein

The protein is present in dairy products and may be used as a supplement to help your body repair tissue as well as burn fat. It's a great food for your body's structure. It's also believed for its ability to boost the immunity compound called glutathione which assists to improve the body's own antioxidant system.

If you're able to detect high levels of glutathione in intense exercise, it will boost the loss of fat and improve your exercise performance.

While you're training sprints make sure you are supplementing with protein from whey on a regular basis. This will boost your metabolic as well as the support for healing of the tissues, and boost antioxidant condition.

Vinegar

Vinegar ensures that the body doesn't conserve carbohydrates as fats instead, but rather as glycogen in muscle. Consuming vinegar as a flavoring for your food can result in a lower the insulin response to carbohydrates as well as improved pancreatic function. It is easy to add vinegar to salads and you'll still get the benefits, and also experience an average increase in blood sugar.

Balsamic and white wine are among the most sweet vinegars, but you are able to utilize any type of vinegar for these great and essential benefits to fat loss.

Eggs

They are an excellent source of protein that contains the optimum amount of choline. It protects your liver from an accumulation of fat. Also, it is a precursor of acetylcholine that is a neurotransmitter that stimulates. The increase in acetylcholine could lead to an increase in the concentrations of the growth hormones that have the power to burn fat.

Eggs can also provide an extra boost to your metabolism thanks to their protein-rich content by their thermogenic effect.

Eggs are chock full of cholesterol, but they don't increase the levels of cholesterol in the bloodstream. The body makes use of the cholesterol found within them to make testosterone. It also improves the effectiveness of the muscle cell membranes.

It is recommended to have eggs at least a few times each week in order to make sure your body is getting more cholesterol and protein consumption.

Kimchi

This is a kind that is a type of Korean food. It is a result of fermentation Napa cabbage onion, garlic, as well as fiber. It's been proven to increase ability to regulate insulin, improve digestion, and enhance the process of losing fat.

An investigation that was conducted recently revealed that if you eat 100 grams of Kimchi throughout the course of one month, you'll shed 1 and 1/2 percent of your body fat. The blood cholesterol and sugar levels will drop by the end of the month.

Coffee

The caffeine in coffee can boost your metabolic rate, resulting it burning calories. Additionally, it aids to shift your body's metabolism to burning fat instead than glucose for the energy needed for its usage. In addition coffee can reduce the chance of developing Alzheimer's, protects the body from damaging oxygen-based species, and can even help regulate blood sugar levels.

There is no definitive study of the importance of coffee on weight loss, but there is a consensus that taking half a cup of coffee daily over a period of a month can cause losing two and a half pounds.

Caffeinated coffee is extremely beneficial as it boosts your performance increasing motivation and vitality. It is the ideal beverage to drink prior to your exercise. It can increase your amount of intensity and capacity of the workout you carry out.

Coffee consumption in conjunction by a healthy and balanced lifestyle and intense training can result in the weight loss and improved the body's composition. Green tea has the same benefits if you don't favor coffee.

Vegetables and Broccoli Cruciferous

If you're looking to reduce the amount of estrogen from the body, ensure that you eat the cruciferous veggies. These include broccoli and cauliflower and removes both naturally produced and chemical estrogens. They contain substances which can connect with genes that are responsible for binding estrogen.

Additionally, they contain high levels of fiber and use them to improve the insulin response of your body, thereby reducing the intake of carbs. They also trigger an extremely controlled response to insulin. This makes them an ideal food to aid in losing fat.

Consuming dark green veggies are also very rich levels of antioxidants. Consuming multiple servings of cruciferous vegetable regularly is the best and most efficient method to follow. If you want to reap maximum benefits, consume them raw. However, should you not feel at ease with cooking them, boil them up and ensure you get at least a portion of vegetables daily.

These foods you've been taught about earlier are designed to aid you in losing fat off your body, and get that toned, beach-body you want to achieve. These are just a few ways they can help the body to accomplish:

I. They in essence increase the usage of fats as energy sources in the body, and not carbohydrates. They helps you shed the fats, and makes you feel more energetic.

II. They make sure that glucose in the blood is utilized to provide fuel source (or stored as glycogen in the muscle) through reducing chronic inflammation as well as increasing the ability of cells to respond to insulin.

III. They assist in burning more energy as breakdown of food takes place by helping the healing of tissues as well as improving your body's resting metabolic speed.

IV. They reduce the feeling of hunger, by boosting leptin and eliminating estrogen excess as well as reducing cortisol and insulinAll this happens by enhancing the response the hormones have to foods.

Chapter 3: Sprinting And Its Effectiveness

If you took one look at the hundred metres sprinters, and those who complete the long marathon - and even run the half marathon, you'd see the advantages from sprinting right away. The majority of sprinters are well-built and have muscles everywhere, while marathoners appear unfitter in comparison.

It is because running in the fastest speed possible and for as long as you are able, you end up leaving your body's metabolism burning calories while toning your muscles. However, the lower intensity exercise that is found in marathons that are long usually makes use of your muscles to help burn the calories and, consequently, you'll lose pounds and muscles within your body.

Studies have demonstrated that short sprint workouts will assist you in losing weight more effectively and without sacrificing the muscle mass. They're far superior to long endurance training the majority of people go because they believe that the harder they work out in a row, the more they'll shed; however, that's not true in a way in that you'll lose the weight as well as your muscles.

Researchers have completed some research and have discovered that short sprints tune the muscles so that they can achieve anabolic levels which allows them to build muscle mass as well as improve the structure of the body. The reason for this is that sprinting has been proven to stimulate the synthesis of protein in your muscles, which can help to prevent the loss of muscle tissue while you work out.

If you're interested in lose weight and get rid of those extra pounds of fats, running is the best method to follow. The endurance training is a different way to draw on your fat reserves, and eventually make their move to the muscles which isn't exactly what you want to begin with.

If you have two people seeking to shed the extra pounds and let one group focus on sprints and intensive workouts while the second group concentrate on endurance training over some time, you'll be able to discover a variety of outcomes.

The team that took part in the short sprinting training is likely to have burnt lots of calories, but the muscle mass will be healthy. It's a tough workout that gives the effect of afterburn that guarantees that your body will be continuing to burn calories even after the training. Your body's metabolic rate increases in order to produce more energy, in order to make sure that muscles are at ease after the exercise. Other endurance training groups is likely to have shed a significant amount of muscle and fat The endurance exercise helps to shed fat however the drawback is because it also consumes the muscles as well.

If your primary aim is losing the extra pounds, your ideal choice is to sprint and intense training. They target the anaerobic energy system that are in your body. They give you the most ideal body composition. If your body is at this ideal state of composition it will allow you to perform activities that require endurance for a long time, like running, soccer, cycling, swimming and running and many more.

How to Do Some Proper Sprinting

What ever you're doing, you need make sure that you do it properly for your desired outcomes. The same is true for sprinting. It is important to do things correctly so that it can work correctly and produce the results that you want. Anything that's going to provide you with good and rapid results isn't going to work out on the field; you will be able to guarantee it.

Here are some suggestions you can follow to ensure that you get all the benefits that the sprint exercise should provide. The only time you will be performing sprints that last around 10 minutes every day. to do that, it is important be able to do it correctly.

Form

A proper form for sprinting is an essential part of the workout. If your form is incorrect, there is a chance of injury. A proper running technique makes you faster. If you're just beginning your run, ensure that your weight evenly distributed between your knees and hands, by placing your knees in a 90 degree angle degrees, and your other knee with an angle between one hundred and a hundred thirty degrees.

In the next step, you must have the power to accelerate when you begin your sprint from the starting location, keep your head lowered while your body is in a straight position until you get to your maximum speed. It is important to elevate your knees at 90 degrees while you run and also your elbows. it's recommended to remain in that position throughout the sprint training.

Get a Proper Running Shoe

It is recommended that you have your feet checked to find out the right pronation in your feet. You want to make sure that you choose a shoe that won't do any injury while running. Whether or not you're under or over pronation is essential that you know this in order to select the correct shoes. Be sure to ensure your shoes run in have been kept dry and never damp in order to perform the job they're necessary to. Make sure to visit the shoe store frequently to make sure you maintain your sneakers in good condition. It is not advisable to buy an old pair of sneakers to utilize it to sprint.

Vary Your Speeds

If you are beginning your workout in a sprint, it's recommended that you take short breaks between. While sprinting, you'll push your body to the max rate that your body is able to manage in a brief amount of time. It is therefore recommended to take a break just a bit in order for your body to replenish itself prior to starting another run. Although it is recommended to have short breaks, be sure you don't allow your heart rate to get returning to its usual rate. Instead, try to reduce it just to a degree before pushing once more.

Rough Terrain

If you plan to race for prolonged lengths of time, it's advised to work out in rough terrain. It will keep the exercise exciting and will ensure that you don't get bored during the course. Make sure the shoe you are wearing has a good grip to ensure that you do not hurt yourself, and you're able to effectively run.

Safety

The sprint exercise is most beneficial when it is done early during the early morning hours to ensure that your metabolic rate is at its peak throughout the throughout the day. This means you'll burn off more calories. However, if you choose to exercise in the evening and go out on the roads, make sure you're wearing reflective clothing in order to prevent accidents from cars that are on the road.

You should push yourself to go at a the speed of one hundred and eighty feet per minute. This may feel weird to you, especially if you're just beginning out but it can be extremely helpful in the end. Make sure you get your feet on the ground smoothly and do not brake when you are on the ground. This brakes could cause injuries to your feet, so be sure to stay clear of that.

If you're not sure that sprinting is the most effective option for you, there are several reasons for why you should pick it up and start with the idea.

Preferential Body Fat Burning

If you're looking to slim down it is essential to ensure that your muscles and bones in good shape. If you choose to sprint for your preferred workout, this will do exactly that to you. It also eliminates the fats that are not needed and gives you the slim body you desire. Training for endurance that is too intense however, will aid in losing everything. the muscles and fats are shed while simultaneously losing fats and muscles and can take longer to lose those.

Eases Access of Body Fat When Needed

This improves the body's metabolism and helps make it simpler for lower intense workouts to utilize the fats needed for energy. Every workout requires energy, even low-intensity workouts. When they aren't able to access fats, they are forced to get the energy they require by burning muscles Sprints make sure that your muscles remain in good shape.

Anabolic

While doing the sprint training, you don't simply burn off hundreds or even tens of calories. You gain the chance to bulk by building muscles, and build the strength. Scientists have studied and have seen the results firsthand.

Mitochondria Building

The function of mitochondria is to draw the energy of nutrients consumed and create ATP that is regarded as the primary source of your body's energy. The process of sprinting can trigger the production of new mitochondria, which implies that it boosts the amount of energy produced by the body. Mitochondria can also be a factor in helping to prevent many of the degenerative illnesses that plague the body. Therefore, it's beneficial having the most healthy mitochondria available inside your body as is possible.

More Effective

You've already realized that sprinting is much superior to endurance exercises. It is less time-consuming than endurance workouts, but it offers many advantages. You will lose many energy by running for around 3 times per week than someone who exercises using endurance training that lasts for 50 to 60 minutes every day.

Going to the Beach

If you're a fan of swimming at the beach, then sprinting is an activity you'll love. In contrast to endurance-training that takes a long time and can be done at the beach is not going to need much effort, sprinting on the beach be more enjoyable and can get harder which means you'll be burning more calories, and the effect of afterburn can last for longer.

Works Great for Overweight People

Sprinting can be a healthful and safe way to exercise, even for obese or overweight individuals. Research has shown that females and males who are obese will benefit from this kind of exercise. This helps them shed weight, increase insulin sensitivity and aids in shedding fat in the hips and around the waist for males.

If you're an overweight individual, take the initiative to ensure that you work out every day for 3 days. It will help get you into excellent shape, and also aid in transforming your body to be fat-adapted.

Seniors should also avoid spending their time doing exercises that are not intense, as they may not be as efficient like the majority of individuals who are trying to shed weight however they'll definitely gain more benefits from it.

Glucose and Insulin

Sprinting as a exercise improves the vital aspects of your body, including sensitiveness to insulin. Also, it reduces postprandial blood glucose response, and can help improve the hyperglycemia of diabetics. This is an exercise that will not simply help in losing weight but also lessens the extent of your disease There's nothing wrong with it.

Blood Pressure

It has the ability to lower high blood pressure. You may experience high blood pressure during a sprint, however at the end of the day, it can help with solving your issue. It is also suitable for sufferer with heart disease or who wants to fix the condition of their heart. Training with high intervals has proved that it is safe for individuals who suffer from heart issues, and there's no need to be concerned about it however it is advisable to talk with your physician before beginning this enjoyable and life-changing experience.

Comes in Different Forms

When it comes to sprinting, many people are only thinking of the 100-meter sprint, but the truth is it is possible to do sprint training in numerous other methods. That includes lifting weights with quick intervals or cycling. It can also include swimming, swimming as well as climbing up hills. The advantages of each are identical and vast, therefore it is not necessary to go running if you hate it. Just find a method that you believe can benefit you.

Chapter 4: Exercise To Accompany Sprints
Have you read about some of the foods
you must eat prior to and during your
workouts so that you can have the body
you've always wanted to look for. In this
section, we'll concentrate on exercises
that you could supplement the sprints you
do to ensure that you reach your goals.

If you examine an elite sprinter, and then
contrast him with an elite marathon
runner there is an enormous difference.
The sprinter's physique which appears to
be designed to look like the shape of a
Spartan soldier, whereas the marathoner
looks more like an ordinary person. This is
due to the exercise form that both man
performs.

For cardio intense interval training, high-
intensity interval training has always been
the top and always has been the ideal
workout to work with.

It is one that combines intervals of intense training like sprinting, but with less intense workouts like walking slow for just a couple of minutes. This type of training is quite different from the steady and slow form of training most individuals are accustomed to.

In this program, you're required to be a runner as that your life is in the balance and it is. One of the benefits is that it will give you higher results in a shorter amount of time.

Exercises that are intense can reduce testosterone levels as well as reduce the immune system's strength and increase cortisol levels and hinder strength gains and halt any hopes of growth. This doesn't mean you shouldn't be able to make the most of strength and muscle growth while working out. This just means you need to be aware of the cardio exercises you do.

Interval Training

The form of exercise was in existence from the late 90s onwards, and plenty of people have gotten amazing physiques by this method of training. It's extremely effective in terms of losing fat and gaining muscle. The primary reason to work out is losing pounds, therefore it's sensible to pick the workout that gives the results you're looking for in the shortest duration of time.

Since its beginnings the interval training has seen a multitude of research studies that have confirmed all of the advantages claimed to be derived from interval training really are.

The training options which will definitely work perfectly with sprinting and aid you in achieving that perfect beach body you're sure to want is:

Barbell Complexes

They've been in use for a long time and have proven to be very efficient. They're very efficient. They can be easily incorporated during your training sessions that are intense particularly at the conclusion or in the beginning, whichever is most suitable for you.

The primary goal of any complex is to build up your body through performing every exercise set at the speed that is most efficient and making sure you use the entire body. Do not speed the exercises as they'll be lost in the process. Each time you complete a complex, you may relax for 60 to 100 and 20 minutes.

Begin with a bar that is empty then gradually increase the weights. be sure to complete the exercises for between eight and 10-minutes.

These are the barbell sets to try:

Total Body Complex

It is similar to the leg day exercise however it includes extra exercises to make this a complete fitness routine for your body.

* Barbell squat

* Squat and push to press

Good morning!

* Romanian dead-lift

* Bent over barbell row

* Power Clean

Lower Body Complex

It is a great final exercise since it does take care not to stress or disturb the unworked parts or part of the body. The moves involved are similar to those performed by your lower muscles.

It encompasses actions like the ones listed below:

* Barbell squats

Good morning!

* Front barbell squats

* Zercher squats

* Romanian dead-lift

Progression of Barbell Complex

The greatest thing about barbells is the fact that they push your body and mind. They shouldn't be a burden each week but be sure to perform them in smaller intervals.

It is easy to add weights to the bar, and increase the number of reps in a set or may gradually cut down the time you rest.

Burpees

It is an excellent kind of workout that you can do without weights. All you require is the space. This is one of the top and most efficient exercises for conditioning in the world. It helps build muscles and aids in burning body fat. The best way to work out is by doing this exercise for between five and ten minutes but no longer.

Burpees Training

If you're trying to stay clear of heavy lifting instead, and focus on more cardio workouts that help burn off some extra fat and build muscle, this workout is that is for you. Begin by performing all the exercises you can within twenty seconds. Then, you take a break every ten seconds and go through the same process throughout the entire time of four minutes.

Total Rep Method

If you're looking for a means that you are able to work yourself harder to achieve a particular standard in your training, then this is a good solution. Create a list of reps you want to complete in 10 minutes. Make sure you reach your goal. Complete the reps, after that, take a rest before doing additional repetitions.

The Two Strongman Intervals

Have you ever wondered why the strongmen tend to be slimmer than other lifters. It's because of the equipment they employ.

* First Set

Start your first exercise by doing many sets as possible in 10 minutes, then you can take a 1 second rest.

Perform both walks of the farmer and sled drag, for approximately fifty metres per set. Then proceed to the next set.

* Second Set

At the same distance of fifty meters, you can work on yoke walks and keg load bearing. The process involves carrying a Keg as well as a yoke for 50 metres.

* Third Set

The third set of exercises must complete the crucifix. This involves lifting yourself using two ropes, tied in a knot to form the appearance of a cross. Perform for thirty seconds. after that, you can move on onto the log lift. complete six repetitions then you're done.

Limit the exercises you do to 3 days per week to avoid overloading your muscles.

It is a fact that we all understand that, at the very least, we think so are aware that prior to starting to work out, it is important to begin by stretching and warming up in order to become fit and ready for the workout. Here are some examples of warm ups and stretching which can aid you in the process.

* Butt Kicks

It will allow you to work your hamstrings as well as strengthen your quads. You should kick your heels until you are able to touch your bottom to pump your arms when you leap and make sure that you remain on your toes.

* High Knee March

While making the knee high marches in the correct way, your posture should be to pump your arms while keeping your feet on the floor throughout the warm up, and then elevating your knees as far as you are able to. Perform this movement for at minimum twenty times.

* Lateral Shuffle

To do this, you'll need to lower your body until your legs are level with the floor and ensure the chest stays elevated. Keep this posture and then quickly shift to the left approximately ten times after which you will shuffle to the same position you began on.

* Cariocas

When you do this, you have to speed up to the side when you cross your left leg that is trailing you then uncross your legs, and shift the leg that is trailing in the back. Continue doing this for a few minutes and build the speed you are moving at each step.

Here are a few warming exercises to assist you to begin your exercise in a safe way that keeps your muscles free of muscle pulls or other related injuries that occur because of a person jumping straight into a workout with no warming up.

The exercises you've been reading about in the article prior to the warm-ups aren't the only ones that could be combined with an vigorous sprinting exercises. There are a variety of the crucial ones to be aware of when you begin to implement the fat-loss program you are working on.

Walking

Training intervals should be performed for shorter durations of time, and walking must be a part of your routine. The intensity of your workouts could be damaging to your health when you fail to make sure that your body is adjusting to the changes. Walking is a great way to relax your muscles as well as improving the heart's health and reducing anxiety.

It is recommended to walk about half-hour per day, or 20 minutes, if you can at all. The interval training and frequent walk each week will make you more lean and muscular, as well as aid in keeping your heart beating.

Chapter 5: The Calories Burning Process And The Amount

Finding out exactly many calories burned when running or sprinting isn't an extremely difficult task. It's just a issue of math. The research has proven that it is possible to lose around one hundred calories every time you race for one mile. The amount of calories that will lose will rise as you increase your the size of your body and the degree to which you're running with less skill or not. This is because you'll need more energy to complete the same distance than an experienced or professional runners. The amount of calories burned doesn't increase when you speed up regardless of how speedy you run. The amount of calories you burn will remain identical.

The calories burnt is only higher when the run is not based on distance but instead on timing; for instance, if you're given 10 minutes to cover as much terrain as you can, you'll certainly cover more than a mile faster, resulting in the burning of more calories. It is estimated that you will consume approximately 5 calories for each liter of oxygen that you breathe in.

A calorie is defined as the amount of energy required to increase the temperature of one kilogram of water by one degree. Calories are determined through the extent to which a person within a calorimetry container warms the surrounding water.

Following a number of research tests, it was evident that there was a definite connection between the amount of oxygen that a person inside the chamber ingested and the quantity of calories his body consumed. The researchers were able to save time since they only required to analyze the amount of oxygen that was inhaled as well as carbon dioxide exhaled.

The technical definition of what we refer as a calorie when doing training is actually 1,000 calories. The term "calorie" was coined due to the usage of kilocalories by using with the same title, however using the Capital "C" at the beginning.

That's why in the event that you are running for a mile, you'll burn around 100 Kilocalories. The amount will vary based on the body's size as well as individual variations and the effectiveness. It is the energy burned in net form as we're burning calories throughout the day even while asleep.

The general rule is that calories per mile is definitely a little different in walking.

In essence, running involves jumping between feet in order to propel your body forward. However, when walking, both feet do not leave the ground. There is bound to be an overlap between extremely fast walking as well as super slow running. Research has shown that walking faster produces more calories than running for the identical distance.

Although you'll burn about the same amount of calories whether you go at a speed or a slow pace for a mile, an fascinating aspect that the majority of individuals are looking for is you will burn different quantities of calories following the race or exercise. If you were running faster, greater the amount of calories you be burning after you're done and running, and not the slow one.

In the following paragraphs, I will explain that there is always the same amount in calories (basal metabolism rate) regardless of the state of inactivity. If you race you, the speed of your heart rate increases as you breathe hard. It isn't recognized by the body's system as being it is resting, and they keep burning fat at high speed until the heartbeats come returned to normal.

If you could consume 7200 calories at eighty percent of maximum VO2max, in contrast the burning of seven hundred twenty calories at a lower sixty percent of your maximum VO2 max, your BMR is increased by 15 to 25 percent, for a entire day. A few other studies fail to provide conclusive figures, however they consistently find that exercising more vigorously can result in a higher and more effective after-burn.

If your primary intention is to shed body fat and shed pounds, you need to consider different options. If you're just beginning, it is recommended to do vigorous sprint exercises at least once each week in order to build up your muscles. In the event of injury, you are at risk that could result in the abrupt end of your exercise. Once you have properly conditioned your body, you'll be able to extend the amount of days you train.

If you are a sprinter, 60 hours of exercise will bring you the same results as an exerciser with low intensity can expect after exercising for 7 hours. If you are a sprinter, 20 minutes of exercise each day can be beneficial as you only have to work long and hard for around 8 minutes due to the small breaks. You will have more advantages over the person who is low-intensity.

In the event that you take part in intense interval training, you'll notice that your body is getting rid of fat in the viscera. you'll see a reduction in waist and notice a decrease in the adipose tissue that is associated with heart issues. This is all possible when you are still eating food at a regular frequency, there is you don't need to alter your eating habits, although it is essential to complement your exercise routine with a nutritious balanced and healthy foods.

Speedy sprinting triggers the body to release high levels catecholamine. It is a class of hormones that trigger the burning of fats to aid in energy production. These hormones are primarily focused on abdominal and visceral fats. A sprint of eight seconds increases your heart rate and simultaneously keeping the release of lactic acid in the right place to stop your muscles from becoming from a rapid fatigue.

Chapter 6: The Low Intensity Workout Misconception

It is likely that you have read the book starting from the beginning and it's time to get rid of the air about the reasons to choose sprinting instead of a less common, low-intensity exercise. It's true that you've likely had a long at the gym or at home performing exercises that are low in intensity to aid in losing weight.

The speed of running can increase energy and fat loss in a small amount of time when compared with workouts that are not as intense. It is a mistake to drive to the gym, running on the treadmill for a jog around all over the place is absurd. Equipment for cardio is exactly identical; they will not provide any kind of motivation since you're only in one spot jogging.

The Misconception

A lot of people enjoy the benefits of workouts that are low-intensity for those who want to shed those excess pounds and achieve that perfect beach body. This is because they are in the search for ways to aid in losing more calories and shed more body fat instead of carbohydrates.

Carbohydrates and fats constitute the main energy source in the body at any time during an task. For carbohydrates, the main consumed energy source is blood glucose. When your body is used completely, it shifts to glycogen that is the storage of glucose.

Then, if you're still working, then the next source of energy soon be fats. It happens after a lengthy duration, such as if you were doing a race or something like that.

Keep in mind that there's always multiple energy sources inside your body at moment. There is always a variety of sources in different proportions, and these are changing over time. The first phase will be the highest amount of carbohydrates, and a lower quantity of fats The two then shift with the fats being consumed greater than carbohydrates.

The idea of less intense workouts burning more fats is because to help the body reduce fats, there's an oxygen requirement. It is believed that the body will have greater oxygen availability as you aren't in a state of exhaustion as opposed when doing intensive exercises like running. The evidence suggests that you'll be burning more fats, but it's much more than.

Most calories burnt is from fat, especially in the case of doing a moderate exercise. However, the problem is that you'll end with burning less calories in all. If you do intense exercises, you'll burn more calories, even though less of them come from fats.

A number of research studies conducted to ensure that the low-intensity workout theory has been put to rest.

The numbers below are not actually the actual figures that are involved in losing calories. They are simply numbers that I thought of to help explain this point in order to reinforce the idea.

For instance, two individuals exercising, one of them using high intensity exercises while the other is doing exercising at a high intensity.

A person who is low-intensity takes sixty minutes for the exercise, which is about 3 miles. Each mile burns a hundred calories. The total time he has burnt three hundred calories.

If we assume that around 60% of calories consumed are from fats (these are fats that circulate in the body) so the person would have burnt approximately 175 calories from fats within the body.

In contrast an athlete who is high in intensity exercising for just 20 minutes in sprints is likely to lose around 600 calories. The person who did this will use more carbs and less fat as energy. If you believe that 40 percent of his energy consumed was from fats the guy would have used around 2400 calories with fat only.

It is evident that when you sprint even for a shorter amount of time, it is more effective in burning calories than a person who does a low intensity training.

The research is showing that even though the majority of us dislike intense training, they're among one of the safest options in terms of burn of numerous calories in a small length of time. Also, you get the post effects of burning that leave your body burning fat once you've finished the workout.

Chapter 7: Definition

Jogging is a continuous forward movement that is performed by legs. The speed of jogging is between running and walking. It is an art form, and jogging is a delicate blend of body movements that are coordinated. In terms of science, this practice improves the anatomy of the body the physiology, psychology, and anatomy.

Jogging, walking, and running all have the similar advantages for health. Running is moving with a lower speed while jogging can be a step ahead and is a lot more intense as compared to walking however it is lesser impact when compared with running. The three exercises when performed frequently can help tone and improve the strength of your muscles, ease tension and increase mood levels and energy levels and, most importantly, reduce the chance of developing high blood pressure, coronary artery disease as well as high cholesterol and the condition known as diabetes. The three exercises have their own advantages and disadvantages. Walking is less calorific as it has a relatively low-impact, it puts less stress on feet and knees. Running or jogging, due to its effect on body can increase the density of bones, however it could result in more injuries. In contrast it burns calories and may eventually bring the loss of weight.

Jogging is a vital part of many athletics. Exercises for training include jogging as well as running. They are performed in a variety of ways in order to improve athletes in endurance, flexibility endurance, and strength.

Chapter 8: Reasons To Consider Jogging

Jogging is an essential form of exercise and training. It is common for athletes to jog during training as it's the fundamental exercise in all sports, and it is the genesis to running. Soccer, basketball, tennis as well as football are just a few of the numerous other sports that require running. If athletes did not run, they are left out because running can help increase endurance. The coach Matt Fitzgerald referred to jogging as a simple form of running "Easy running is great because the more of it you do, the fitter you get, and because it's not terribly taxing you can do a lot of it." It is said that Arthur Lydiard defined it as, "Stamina, not strength can produce the necessary condition of unstoppableness that is the mark of a most fit and healthy person. Stamina refers to the ability for continuous work, which is achieved through the general training of the cardio-respiratory system, and the systematic building up of muscles generally." It is now clear the reasons why and how jogging can be included in the routine of athletes and it's due to running that they're able to maintain their focus on their activities.

Another motive for people to consider exercising is for physical fitness. It is a comprehensive method of balancing fitness, nutrition and exercise as well as the need for relaxation. The physical and aerobic exercise is designed to reduce the body's fat levels, constructing muscle mass, shedding pounds as well as achieving the ideal BMI. (BMI). It is not necessary to be jogging, but it can comprise core workouts as well as strength and aerobic activities apart from running and jogging. The desire to become physically fit comes from an awareness of the dangers to health that come from being physically inactive or more of the time, people have suffered from ailments that could have been curable through exercising. It is this realization that makes many take to running to improve their the health of their family members. Inactivity and physical inactivity are the root cause for a number of chronic ailments.

People who exercise are often doing it in order to shed weight. The rise in overweight and obesity can be due to the growing use of internet-based gaming, computers and television, as well as increasing demand for fast food outlets. According to the World Health Organization (WHO) statistics and facts indicate that, in the year 2008, people who were between the ages of 20 and over had 35% of them overweight, and 11% overweight. Based on WHO data, the prevalence of excess weight and obesity ranks 5th in the top risk of deaths worldwide and causes the deaths of around 2.8 million people each year. WHO is also estimating at 44% people who suffer from diabetes as well as 23% of those who suffer from heart disease, and 7 - 41 percent of people who suffer from cancers due to obesity and overweight. In the year 2011, WHO further stated that more than 40 million kids aged five and under were obese and attributed this to eating of foods high in fat as well as physical lack of exercise. Being overweight and obese pose risks to diabetes, hypertension and heart disease. Physical fitness is a factor that goes together with weight loss or control. One of the key factors to losing weight is the increased expenditure of calories over intake of calories. You must keep in mind that calories are required to be able to exercise. It is essential to possess the right quantity and the correct type of fuel available to help the machine operate. It would be best to consult a dietitian/nutritionist on dietary instructions. The benefits of running, both physical and mental, that are described in a different chapter reduce the risk of obesity, excess weight, as well as their risk.

Jogging can be a basic type of exercise since it's easy to perform and can be completed at any time and from anywhere. There is no set of rigid and clear regulations. There is no time to run, and it is an inexpensive physical exercise. An excellent pair of sneakers as well as the proper attire is sufficient for both indoors and outdoors. If indoors the treadmill is utilized however there are advantages as well as disadvantages. It is not necessary to endure bad weather while using a treadmill, and it can make running much easier and more efficient due to the belt that helps in transferring your leg However, it offers the least amount of resistance. Many people find running on the treadmill boring since it doesn't afford a beautiful perspective, however some remain occupied by watching the latest movie. This can also distract you from the task at hand; it keeps you away from looking at the timer from time-to- the time. Many prefer to run in the city, on the street, since they like seeing the hustle and bustle. Others prefer to be in a natural environment that has parks and trails because of the clean air and absence of polluting. These are great places to run. Other people look for areas with scenic views such as bridges and beaches. Ovals for running tracks are often popular because distances can be calculated and the track's surfaces are more comfortable to knees. Others don't care about the place they travel to, and prefer to go wherever they want.

Jogging can tone muscles, particularly the quads, hamstrings, glutes, hip flexors and calves. It is achieved through repetition of movements as well as the use of weights. It is a sport which puts the majority of your muscles in action.

Running can reduce stress. The body's stress response is to stimuli which threaten to destroy our environment. Stressors that are common include stressful jobs as well as job-related uncertainty, bad time management, inability to manage work and family obligations as well as financial pressures and difficulties in communities. When we are under pressure the levels of cholesterol and blood sugars are elevated, and this leads to the development of high blood pressure. The high blood pressure can lead to diabetes, atherosclerosis, and the list goes on and on. Many people like to run at work in order to relieve anxiety. Some say that a change of the scenery is all they require and fresh air or that aftershock feeling that it gives them a relief from all the pressures that are caused by workplace stress. Exercise improves moods, and helps reduce anxiety and depression.

Certain cities offer run tours. They are a enjoyable way of seeing the city. It is possible to arrange the tour depending on the tour route, languages of tour guides and the pace of the group. It blends three of your most-loved activities such as sightseeing, jogging and people.

Many people exercise because they're conscious of the advantages that jogging can bring. They wish to live a healthy life through living a healthy lifestyle. They're one of the very few people who take the time to exercise and balance the exercise with a healthy diet and have the ability to cope with the demands of working.

Some jog as they're urged by friends. They are enthralled by having fun with friends. They also take part in fun runs or marathons. They bring a lots of joy to running.

Chapter 9: Types Of Jogging

Recovery Jog

A recovery jog could also be described as an easy to jog. It is running without putting in any effort or putting in. This helps to boost your distance without working to a high level and can be done immediately following an intensive running session. The recovery jogging routine not only helps your body recover but manage stress during training as well as running quantity. Long runs with high intensity create stress for training, and any time that the body goes through strain, it will eventually exhaust and fatigue. However, when you do these jogging sessions, your body is taught not to quit, but to withstand which in turn leads to exhaustion and fatigue. It is the volume of running that you gain from your the recovery jog, so you are able to be able to run at a slower speed but still have the energy to run for a long time. Writer, coach, as well as nutritionist Matt Fitzgerald suggests that if you are running more than five times per week, your recovery jogs must be incorporated into your schedule to help balance the amount of running and stress from training. Since he doesn't recommend running for long distances within 24 hours after training, an intense exercise, the recovery jog must follow with an 1:1 ratio. For athletes who are training twice per day, the first time must be intense followed by an exercise to recover. When you are recovering, run for as long as you are able and slowly, while preserving your energy for your next exercise.

Base Jog

Jogging for base is running at your normal speed. The speed you run will vary based on your personal preferences as natural paces vary for every person. The weight, height and build affect your speed. While doing jogging that are a bit faster, you must find yourself in your comfortable zone sufficient to work the entire body and perform in an aerobic level. It shouldn't be too difficult This is your normal week-long workout routine. It increases the endurance of your muscles and increases distance.

Long Run

Long runs are designed for endurance purposes, those are the base runs which run longer and aim at putting the runner through a workout. In order to determine if you're prepared for competitions, run long runs to determine whether you can last enough.

Progression Run

Progression runs begin with the pace of natural running and finish by gaining a higher, but moderately difficult speed. The intensity for these runs remains within the aerobic range and is within the base run and the lactate threshold. Progression runs are classified into three subtypes:

* Fast-finish progression run

* Threshold progress

* The Marathon Pan progression

Speed-finish progression runs are those which have a slower first segment followed by a faster second segment. However, this second section is very short with a distance of between one and three miles. It's like preserving your energy in order to endure throughout the entire run. If you're already tired from the initial segment, this second one will be difficult.

Threshold's progression runs include an extended warm-up followed by the speed at which it is possible to run for an hour, or "lactate threshold". When you run this way the body is forced to test the limits of your body. It is a great workout to prepare for marathons.

Progression runs at marathon pace have the advantage of a longer and faster second section, but it is slow compared to earlier discussed run progression.

Fartlek

Fartlek Fartlek is a training program created through Swedish trainer Gosta Holmer. It refers to "speed play" because it is a mix of speedy and hard running of various lengths, speeds and at irregular intervals. The participant should be working within 60to 80 percent of their maximum heart rate. The goal of this type of exercise is to build fatigue resistance and efficacy.

Hill Repeats

Hill repetitions are shorter distances in upward-facing runs to improve aerobic endurance and build resistance to intense fatigue, increase endurance and pain tolerance during the entire run. Hill repeats are performed once you've built endurance and toned your muscles.

Tempo Run

Tempo runs run with the intensity that is known as "lactate threshold". It is the quickest you are able to go without putting yourself into anaerobic strain. The speed of this run can be defined as "comfortably hard". It is the speed at which highly fit athletes are able to go to the top of their speed for at the least one hour, and for novice athletes, it should be at the minimum of 20 minutes. This is aimed at increasing the speed, and then sustain it for a longer period of time.

Interval

Interval training is a series of brief, fast running that is followed by vigorous recuperations. It helps runners include fast runs during an exercise, in contrast to doing it all in a single intense effort that will eventually exhaustion. The process of pushing yourself beyond your maximum and then recovering, increases the body's metabolism as well as its effectiveness. It forces the body to use both the oxygen and anaerobic system. Since it involves both the aerobic and anaerobic system, this increases endurance for the cardiovascular system.

Aqua jog

A different type of jogging involves aqua jogging. It is sometimes called water running. It is typically used by athletes, joggers as well as marathon runners who have suffered injuries caused by. Aqua-jogging is a brand new way to exercise aerobically using the same muscles with not requiring any weight it is a softer approach to knees, feet as well as the hips and the back. Jogging on the water is available in two varieties:

* Jogging through the depth without the feet touching the depths of the pool.

* Jogging in water that is shallow where the feet touch to the surface of the water

Running with feet that aren't touching the depths of the pool must be performed at the bottom and this type of form does not have any impacts and is advised from Ben Greenfield, triathlete and coach. Running in shallow water can be weight bearing, but it has less impact. Shoes for water are required to complete this workout, the purpose of this exercise is to be performed under the water. This helps to increase the intensity of exercise by about 2-3 times than running with in bare feet. It also gives adequate resistance. The use of running shoes in a swimming pool is not permitted as it has also been found to be heavy, sloppy and doesn't create an effortless motion. Running with your feet bare on the pool floor does not generate enough force. In order to stay the water afloat, a floating belt is required to hold the upper part of your body above water, so you will not have to struggle to stay in the water.

Aqua jogging demands a distinct style of exercise compared to conventional running. The body has to be leaning towards the front, and exaggerate your jogging, and bring your knees closer towards the chest, then push back using a wide range of motion while closing your fists, move the arms like the way you do when running.

Chapter 10: Benefits Of Jogging

Physical Benefits

Jogging is an exercise which, when performed regularly, makes every organ of the body function effectively. The effects from jogging regularly have proven positive outcomes.

Aerobic exercise focuses on enhancing cardiopulmonary fitness, making the heart work efficiently by making it stronger and pumping increased oxygen. Regular jogging, as well as other aerobic activities boost the activity of hormones and enzymes in the heart's muscles that allow it to contract efficiently. The ability of the heart to contract is evident by an incredibly low heart rate at rest as well as a high stroke volume, which enhances ability of the blood to transport oxygen. Research has shown that when the heart pumping effectively and the whole cardiovascular system is in good health due to an increase in HDL cholesterol (good cholesterol) and lower LDL cholesterol (bad cholesterol) and low levels of triglycerides and body fat levels as well as improved blood pressure and thinning of platelets which reduces the risk of arrhythmias. Chances of avoiding a heart attack or the possibility of surviving one is increased.

The immune system can also benefit when you exercise regularly. Infectious diseases can be prevented due to the increase in immunoglobulins. Running also stimulates white blood cells production, which assists in fighting off illnesses. Another way is to battle infections and various other illnesses.

Through jogging, more efficient digestion as well as improved the function of bowels are attained.

Running improves endurance of muscles, as you do more regularly, is the better muscles are taught to not tire quickly. The endurance that ordinary joggers, runners and athletes have cultivated that allows them to work consistently, but retain the strength to perform other tasks.

Jogging can also be effective to burn off unwanted fat. When you jog regularly, approximately 3-4 times per week, your metabolism will be raised and, as a result the increased metabolic rate the calories will also be burned quicker.

As jogging can be a highly impact-inducing sport the bone density increases particularly in the back, leg joints, and hips. Thus strong bones develop to prevent osteoporosis. An analysis of the impact of running to increase bone mass found that men who exercised nine or more each month, had greater bones mass density than men who exercised between one and eight every month. In the same study, researchers also discovered that jogging can increase levels of bone mass on the femoral neck, also known as the thigh's neck bone. The flexibility of joints can also be increased and helps reduce the chance of injuries.

The body's ability develops to sleep more peacefully and relax when you run; it's an effective treatment for insomnia and chronic fatigue.

Jogging is a great exercise that extends your longevity. In the EuroPRevent 2012 the Dr. Peter Schnohr of the European Society of Cardiology presented new data through the Copenhagen City Heart Study and He confirmed the effects of exercising. Dr. Schnohr stated that regular jogging improves the lifespan of men by 6.2 years, and 5.6 year for females. smoking cigarettes shortened the life span by 9 years. The researcher further said that since it is a strenuous sport, it doesn't require a daily commitment for the duration of one to two and a half hours each week spread over two to three times, is sufficient for maximum benefit, particularly when it is done at a slower to moderate pace. This research began in the year 1976 and involved twenty thousand people and women. The nature of the disease was examined when a large number of participants died in the initial six years, and also observational trials were conducted too.

Psychological Benefits

The endorphins produced by the pituitary gland in lengthy, as well as moderate to intense exercises. They can cause "runner's high", a sense of wellbeing. Analgesia can also be a consequence from endorphin release since they are able to bind with the receptors that cause pain. Additionally, they act as stimulant, and that's why when you exercise regularly, your capacity to relax increases and better sleeping patterns are established. The fact is, it's through endorphins, moods improve as is the feeling of pain less and stress levels are reduced, and anxiety and depression are prevented from occurring. For anxiety and depression, running has demonstrated to be an effective treatment, but it isn't used regularly. Since endorphins can be produced by our bodies, joggers aren't dependent on them. The regular exercise routine produces higher levels of endorphins. Keeping to your routine is simple in the end as people are able to find the incentive to run as it induces feelings of euphoria, as well as "runner's high"

The "runner's high" produces results. People who run gain confidence during their training. If you're confident, you're motivated to push yourself harder and conquer any hurdle that is thrown at you. Also, when you feel confident due to the loss of weight. It guarantees that you're doing the right thing since you experience a surge in self-esteem. This is the reason the fact that runners are more productive at work; they are able to manage the stress of running. They discover a method to overcome their issues by jogging. They are able to relieve their anger by running. They can improve their self-esteem by jogging. It does this due to the fact that your body operates at an aerobic level which means that the requirement for oxygen is very high. once it is in the brain, it is able to function better. It results in a clearer mental focus as well as improved memory and learning.

Yes, there are drugs available to help with anxiety and depression however, since it is an activity that is natural that can aid in treating anxiety and depression. Running helps lower levels of cortisol and adrenaline these chemicals which are responsible for anxiety. Additionally, it helps distract your mind to stressors that cause anxiety. It is the reason why people who jog prefer to go outside because it clears their attention off the things that are bothering them.

A study conducted by the University of Texas Southwestern Medical Center in 2005 showed the symptoms of depression decreased by nearly half after 30 minutes of physical activity that was moderately challenging five days per week.

Chapter 11: Prepare To Start

Get medical approval from your physician of family origin A physical exam will identify the state of your health. If you think that you're physically healthy taking a baseline health exam could help. It's important to see your physician regardless of age, particularly in the event that any of these applies to you:

If you are older than 65 and you do not engage in exercise.

If you have heart disease, it is likely that you are at risk.

* You live a life of sedentary living

Are you either obese or overweight.

If you smoke or you have stopped smoking cigarettes

If you have hypertension, it is likely that you are

* If you suffer from diabetes.

* The history of your family may include heart disease and diabetes

* You experience chest pains

If you experience dizziness, or fainting

There was an accident that you suspect could have an impact on you.

Set your intentions and plans with your doctor. He may conduct a series of tests. He might discuss possible issues. When you're cleared you are able to begin.

Warm Up and Cool Down

It's important to get warm before you start jogging or running. Why? The best way to warm up is by ensuring the optimal results from physical exercise by slowly dilating blood vessels, which increases the rate of heart beat, respiratory speed, and circulation of blood within the muscles.

The body is communicating to your heart that it needs to get ready for a faster pumping rate, sending it a quick note will not do the body any favors. The warm-up also relaxes muscles as well as opens joints. The proper warm-up helps prepare the body to be able to perform and reduces the chance of injury.

Warm-ups last for a certain amount of time according to the intensity of the exercise. This gives your body an opportunity to introduce its intended activity. The process of warming up the muscles in the lungs can increase the volume of your lungs, and increase your respiration rate and allow for adequate supply of oxygen.

The warm-ups boost the body temperature to allow for maximum flexibility and effectiveness. They help get your muscles prepared. Concentrate on working key muscles to include those in the hamstrings, glutes and arches and calves of the feet. The key is to begin slowly, and don't try to speed up your pace.

The warm-up process takes between 10 and 20 minutes. It should correspond to the duration and intensity of the fitness routine. Warm-up exercises are performed in order to get your heart ready to increase its pumping speed. What is the speed? Note the resting heart rate. run at a moderate pace, slowly the heart rate up to Zone 1, then Zone 2, at the point that you are sure you are ready to go to go on, you can move into Zone 3 for about two or three minutes. The target heart rates and zones will be covered in the identical chapter. It will provide you with some idea of whether you're doing enough.

The next step is to perform active warm-ups. They are also known as dynamic stretching, they can help stretch your muscles. Dynamic warm-ups are stretching exercises that are performed while moving. However those stretches that most of us have come across are static, and do require the body to shift from one position to the next. The intensity of the warming up depends on age and health of the person who is jogging. Work out with the both the upper and lower body. Then gradually increase your intensities. Here are some quick warming exercises that work on every muscle engaged in jogging.

Jogging is easy and takes 10-20 minutes.

* Take a walk on your toes and hold them for 30 minutes. This helps increase ankle movement, strengthening muscles of the calves, as well as improving balance.

* The arm can swing. The swings help increase the range of motion in your shoulder, maintaining a 90 degree angle of

elbow. Begin slowly, then slowly increase speed, as the range of motion grows.

* Hug your arm. Do this for 10 to 15 minutes and then repeat it at least twice. It helps improve shoulder flexibility.

* Arm circle. The exercises are based on flexibility also. At first, you should extend your arms outwards and turn slowly. Begin with tiny circles. Gradually expand the radius of the circles. Repeat this on each side and over a period of 30 minutes.

Straight leg kicks. It actively warms the hip flexors and hamstrings and increases stabilization of the core. Maintain a straight back as you stand up tall and lift one leg in a row, keeping the knee straight. With the your ankle flexed. Then, with the hands to the opposite leg's side, try to reach the feet. Do the exercise for about 10 minutes, then switch legs and perform the same exercise with the opposite leg. Repeat this twice.

* Swings of the legs. This helps increase the hip motion. The legs should be swung between front and back and maintain a straight posture. Perform this for 30 minutes for each leg.

* Walk with a high knee. Walking at a normal speed, bringing the knee back up. This will help enhance the hip's flexion. Keep the knee in the middle of your body to the highest point it is possible while keeping your opposite foot positioned on the tiptoe.

* Butt kickers. This helps to stimulate the Hamstrings. Begin by running forward, but then the legs should be pushed up towards the back.

* Forward lunge. This stimulates the glutes. Lean forward, with your feet firm on the floor, keeping your knee and hip to

the same level as your feet. Maintain the body upright.

It's equally important to know if the workout that you're doing is sufficient, appropriate and/or too much. Examine how much effort you've performed and a concrete method of determining if you're doing enough work is measuring your heart rate target. The target heart rate is the level that, if it is it is sustained, you are believed to be secure and efficient. This guide is an excellent one for you to follow if you wish to understand how to perform your exercise.

The first step is to determine the resting heart rate of your body by measuring your heart rate at the beginning of your morning prior to getting out of your bed or doing anything. The typical heart rate ranges between 60 and 80 beats per minute. When you're active and physically fit and are not in a hurry, their resting heart rates typically lower as their heart muscles are able move blood more efficiently.

The next step is to find the highest heart rate. This is the most heart-beat rate that could be achieved by the heart, without issues and is dependent on your age.

Studies on how to determine maximal heart rates is numerous, and several of formulae were derived from various research studies and claim to be the best measure of heart rate maximum. The most popular formula was developed created by Professor. William Haskell and Dr. Samuel Fox because of its simplicity in calculation and retaining. It is also used by the American Heart Association uses this formula as well.

* To determine, MHR = 220 times your age.

* The ideal heart rate ranges from 50% to 85 percent of your heart rate.

At any point during exercising, you should check the pulse of your wrist with two fingers: your forefinger and middle finger. Also, you can examine your carotid pulse.

*You can choose to keep your pulse counted for 10 seconds before multiplying by six. The whole minute of counting can disrupt your daily routine, and it's difficult to manage when you're running. Many joggers carry an electronic heart rate gauge. On both occasions will allow you to see if you're in the range of your heart rate target.

Let's dissect the distinct heart rate zones.

* Zone 1. Healthy Heart Zone -- The zone lies within 50-60 percent of your maximum heart rate. It is also the most simple to reach. Here is where the warm ups begin. By taking a fast walking, you'll

have the ability to boost the heart rate up to the range of. If you aren't able to engage in high impact workouts in this range, maintaining it can be beneficial. Brisk walking with low-impact may reduce body fat levels and blood pressure and reduce cholesterol. There is a claim that 85percent of calories consumed in this area originate from fats. There is no age limit to get active. Walking falls within this area and also has many benefits.

* Zone 2 Zone 2, Fitness Zone It is a zone that lies within 60-70% of your maximum heart rate. The result of your efforts here is exactly the same like that in zone 1. But, the majority of calories burned come result from fat, and this is why it is referred to as the fat burning zone.

* Zone 3. Aerobic Zone The Aerobic Zone zone lies within 70 to 80 percent of the heart's maximum rate. The functions that your heart as well as your respiratory

system are strengthened. It is the place where your heart is doing its job and your lung muscles are at more intense rate to accommodate the demands of oxygen. The strength and size of the heart is increased in the process, which means that it's pumping capacity increases. This is the ideal zone for the endurance exercise. Fats calories remain burning, but at a 50percent level.

* Zone 4. Anaerobic Zone * Zone 4, Anaerobic Zone zone is located within 70-80 percent of the heart's maximum rate. It is the area of the training for performance. It is where athletes train since it boosts the VO2 maximum. Vo2 max refers to the highest achievable amount of oxygen in the body is able to absorb. Within this zone it is close to its highest levels, but even at the highest intake of oxygen, it's insufficient to meet the requirements of the muscles in the heart's. Heart function

is deficient in this situation as it's now in the anaerobic zone Acidosis is on the way to increase. It is good to know that it is possible to train the heart to perform at this rate and the lactate tolerance can be enhanced. With proper instruction and supervision an endurance of this degree can be built. The fat is still burning in this area, but it is only 15%.

* Zone 5 Red Line -- This zone lies within 90-100 percent of the heart's maximum rate. The zone that is most intensive. Training with high intensity requires you to reach and maintain the zone for between 30 and 60 minutes. There is a possibility that working at this level can lead to the burning of muscles.

Beginners should start slowly through warm-up exercises in Zone 1. Gradually move to Zone 2. keep your heart rate in the zone for about 20 minutes If you are feeling that it's getting too intense, don't take it too seriously, and go back in zone 1 to rest. Protect your muscles from injuries while letting the muscles be prepared for exercise the following day. Keep track of the intensity of effort so that you can get an idea of the extent to which you're working hard.

If you feel that the five zones are too complex there is a second way to comprehend the how to deal with the intense. This book's goal is to educate novices, and serve as a guidance to reach the objectives established. Intensity levels for exercises:

* Exercise lightly -- 40-45% of your maximum heart rate

Exercise moderately 50% to 60% of the maximum heart rate. Fat is being burned up at this point.

* Exercise vigorously is 70 to 85% of the maximum heart rate is performed at a high aerobic rate

The 5 zones and intensities levels can help you determine how to achieve the goals you have set. With each level an individual goal could meet whether it's fitness or weight loss, burning fat or prepare for a contest. For a reminder, don't not do too much exercise; you must take note of your body. It is suggested to begin by doing a minimum of 30 minutes a day, or 150 minutes every week.

While a warm-up is essential to begin a exercise, a cooling down is just as important for the end of a run. Cooldowns help the body gradually transition from a strenuous training session to a more relaxed state. This will gradually bring the heart back to an unwinding state. The circulation of blood from the heart to muscles during training, and upon back, the muscle-skeletal pump aids in the return of venous blood towards the heart. A brief pause during the training can cause the blood volume to be large trapped in peripheral veins and the heart racing quickly and the volume of blood. Not enough oxygen gets distributed to the body. As a result it is stressful for the heart and joggers may experience the sensation of being dizzy. A cooling down process reduces the risk of fainting and dizziness for experienced runners or joggers.

Stretching statically is great to cool down, and helps to prevent tightness of the muscles as well as prevent injuries. Do some stretching exercises on the muscles employed.

It is important to gradually reduce the amount of energy you expend during the jog or run. These are some cool-down activities you can do following exercise.

* Run slowly for about 10 minutes, then take a brisk stroll.

* static stretching. Do gentle stretches.

• Stretch your quadriceps muscles by pulling the heel of your left towards the glute of the left Hold for about 10 seconds, then repeat the exercise on the opposite leg. Repeat this 2-3 times.

• Stretch your hamstrings. In a supine posture, straighten the leg, then raise it above the hips. Then, grip your calf or thigh and keep it for 10 to 15 seconds, then perform the same exercise for the opposite leg. Repeat this 3 times.

• Stretch your glutes. In a supine posture then bend the knee of your left and then cross the right leg across it. Lower the left knee towards the chest and keep it there for about 10 minutes. Repeat the exercise three times.

* Extend your chest. Connect fingers around the neck. Straighten out arms simultaneously gazing upwards. Repeat the exercise a couple of times.

* Extend the triceps as well as shoulders. Straighten both arms then bend both joints at the elbow and then extend your left hand to the mid-back then gently pull the left elbow by using the other hand. Use the left arm to carry across your chest and gently push the elbow until it begins to make it extend past the shoulder. Change arms.

The back should be stretched. Place yourself on your fours Round your back. Then reverse it to form an L-shape by putting your spine in. Repeat the exercise three times.

* Hydrate. Refill electrolytes and fluids which were depleted. This helps reduce

muscle pain and help improve the flexibility and strength.

• Drink a glass of chocolate milk or a protein shake. Proteins and carbohydrates must be replenished.

* Massage. Following an intense exercise, think of that your muscles are tired, and a massage can aid in recovery and relaxation of muscle tension.

Cooldowns must be slow but never stop so that you can slow down such as from a run into a jog and then an easy walk. If you've jogged with a moderate level, stretching and walking are a great way to cooling down.

Attire

Shoes

The feet propel your body when you jog, and they absorb the force, which can be as high as three to two times body's weight.

Also, the feet stand between your body and the surface, so the more hard the surface is, the more difficult the impact on knees, feet as well as the back. If the surface is smooth, such as grass, it's less prone to injury for the knees, feet, and back. For those who are just beginning, it's crucial to choose footwear that is comfy and reduce the impacts. When choosing the appropriate footwear, the biomechanics of both feet need to be assessed. The first step is to determine what the characteristics that your strike. Also, find out the way each foot is placed on the floor. There are three varieties of foot strikes which include neutral foot strike as well as overpronated, as well as supinated feet strike.

In the neutral foot strike The heel first lands and then the mid-foot after which there's an arch flattening (rolling inside) which is followed by a forward foot strike, which rolls across the arch before finishing by pushing off. The most important aspect of this form of striking is the lowering of the arch. It is referred to as pronation because that is where the impact absorbs. For people with neutral fees the shoe of your choice will do so in the event that it's comfortably.

The strike of the overpronated foot occurs caused by excessive mid-foot roll. to the side and fails to let out as it should in the time of the release. It is common among flat feet, and is often the cause of to injuries from excessive use. For people with pronated feet take care to wear footwear with strong midsoles.

In contrast when you strike your feet supinated, the arch flattens and the foot doesn't slide in. The outer foot is able to absorb the shock. If you have supinated feet, put on footwear that is well cushioned and elastic.

Consider the kind of foot you've got. A second aspect to take into consideration is the structure, build and the mass that your physique. If you are jogging for a long time, your heels as well as the mid-foot are subjected to the highest load. It is advised to find adequate cushioning in the mid-foot and heel to ensure optimal assistance. A good pair of shoes will help keep you safe from injury and injuries. For jogging shoes wear them later at night when your feet are expanding. Select shoes that can be flexed towards the front foot to allow for the expansion and bend of your toes when you push them off. There must be room for your toes to stretch. There are occasions when feet have different dimensions. Choose footwear based on the dimensions of the foot that is larger.

It is also recommended to replace your shoes following 500 to 400 miles of jogging, or running as the shoes will not absorb the shock properly in the first 500 miles.

It is currently unclear what the heel strike patterns is superior to midfoot strike patterns. Experts are constantly debating regarding this matter. Although minimalists believe that forefoot strike is more effective.

Socks

Socks are just as important as shoes. They are essential to be comfortable to be able to do your job. Avoid solely cotton socks as they are prone to soak up sweat, causing blisters. Select socks composed of acrylic and polyester since they absorb moisture. To keep winter cold, choose socks that are made of wool-based blends, or double-layer socks.

Shirts

Choose comfortable clothes for jogging. To stay dry you should wear fast-wicking shirts that will keep you dry during your workout and assist in controlling the body's temperature. Additionally, consider wearing loose-fitting clothing to allow for greater fluidity.

Women, it's recommended to put on a sports bra since it provides support for breasts and helps reduce discomfort, by flattening the breasts and limiting movements. Bras for sports can also be worn by males with big breasts, for the same reason just as women wear them.

Running Shorts

The running shorts you wear should be comfortable and swiftly wicking away sweat and avoid the chaffing. The running shorts come with liners, they don't need to put on underwear. If you aren't a fan of shorts for running and are searching for something different, you should look at shorts that can retain moisture and are air-conditioned. Avoid wearing cotton or nylon as they easily soak up sweat and create the chaffing.

Running Tights

The tights that run on the muscles, shield against the cold and heat, as well as against water (sweat or rain) as well as being aerodynamic.

Chapter 12: Correct Jogging Techniques
Right Form

A proper jogging posture is essential to maximise the benefits of exercising for the body and minimize the chance of sustaining injuries. You must look in the direction of your eyes and keep the head straight, and not tilting or looking downwards or letting the head slide. Maintain your body in a straight line for maximum breathing. This will help relax facial muscles. Relieve your shoulders when you feel that your shoulders are tense Give it a the range of motion exercise to loosen the muscles and help conserve the energy. Maintain your knees at a low angle. Make sure arms are close to your body. Let arms move, but stay at a low level, then relax and keep the elbows to 90 degrees allow arms to swing outward however, not toward the midline, to reduce the rotation of the torso. Do not place arms too close to the chest. Holding arms closer to the body will cause tension and tightness in the neck and shoulders. Hold your hands in a cup, but do not build a fist, and hold it tightly, just keep your hands loose. Make sure to lean back when you move so that you distribute weight equally to every foot. Jumping too far will make you fall in a tense manner, causing more impact.

There is a constant controversy over the question of foot strike, namely whether it is the heel strike, or mid-foot strike is more effective. The reality is that most runners and athletes land on their heels. It is a natural thing, but research shows that it causes greater injuries to knees as well as hamstrings, shins and knees. Mid-foot strikes provide greater shock absorption, and places less stress on Achilles tendon as well as the calves. Also, it avoids the need for shin bandages. Since every person is different so one approach may not be suitable for others. Make sure you choose a foot move that you're at ease in and can prevent injuries too.

It's commonplace to run in the street, but it's not advised to run in the street every day. Take a break from your body by running on areas with soft surfaces. This can reduce the pressure on your knees, feet and the hips. Explore other surfaces like grass, sand or trails. An investigation found that grass has 17% less stress on feet. A softer surface can give knees and feet the chance to rest for a short period of time. The risk of injury decreases.

Running on different terrains may need different forms.

The upward incline of jogging will help burn off more calories, increase oxygen supply, and is beneficial in the gym as the jogger is quicker and faster. The muscles in the legs are strengthened, giving greater strength and endurance. Based on the slope and the slope, you can adjust the size of your knees. You can also shorten your stride while at while increasing your speed. Make sure you land at the middle of your gravity, and slightly in front of your leading foot. The pumping of your arms to your stride. The longer you run, the steeper the gradient the more this arm movement will encourage you to overcome gravity and the hill, but make sure you keep safety in mind. Some would be able to conquer the hill with no cost Be aware that the advantages from jogging can be enjoyed if you exercise for the for a long time. Beware of accidents.

Running downhill is a completely different style. When gravity pulls you downwards the body is exposed to greater impact, aided by the weight of your body. There is a risk of the quadriceps or knee injury.

Place your feet on your feet's heels or in the middle of your foot, don't lean to the side and use your feet as brakes. follow the gravity with the speed that you are able to control.

Though most people just run around the neighborhood with their roads made of concrete to more challenging locations or types of terrain It is important to try different kinds of surfaces and terrains. Running on concrete or asphalt isn't recommended as the surfaces offer almost zero shock absorption to the feet and can result in more risk of injury. Running on sand or grass trails, or hills on other hand, allows one to adapt quickly and increase physical fitness. Different terrains can also bring diverse challenges, which result in an entirely new workout routine for muscles. The workouts lead to increased muscular strength and eventually quicker jogging technique. When you jog on the correct surface, the risk of injury can be reduced and result in an enjoyable jogging experience. Gorgeous scenery is among advantages of shifting your "jogging" area. Beaches are commonly used as locations for jogging, especially those looking to work out with water and sand, as well as parks for those looking to experience jogging on hills, grass, or trails, offer the chance to connect with the natural world. Here are a few well-known terrain types as well as what can joggers do to enhance their the training they can get from these terrains:

* Grass: The most comfortable place to run in is grass it has about 17 percent less pressure on your feet while jogging in grass compared to the concrete roads. It is due to the ability of grass's surface to absorb any footfalls. It also features an uneven surface. It's a good thing because it forces you to work your leg muscles.

However, it can cause instability. The result could be injuries to your ankles and ligaments. It is ideal for testing your speed. It's much more enjoyable to speed up on grass, or quickly jog before slowing down to your usual jogging pace.

* Sand - Jogging on sand is commonly associated with the beach, is difficult for many despite it being among the most soft terrains. The reason is that it is uneven, and moves on impact. It is essential to keep your legs moving so that they don't sink into the sand. The benefit is that it could result in more aerobic activity, which results in higher calories being burned (about 1.6 times greater than normal running) However, this increases the risk of damage as changing levels of sand can make it more difficult to sustain knee and ankle injury. Sand running is not advised for people suffering injured or have weak ankles due to the additional stress that

sand causes on legs. If you can train closer towards water the more beneficial because the sand is thicker and offers an increased grip. Make sure to switch between dry sand as well as the soft sandy sand, to test your skills.

• Trails: Dirt tracks are a the perfect opportunity to be in touch with the natural world. Working with roots and rocks aids in focusing and focus on their exercise and encourages you to exercise better control and balance. Running on trails that are dirt can reduces the pressure to your foot. They also offer plenty of opportunities to work out on hills, usually with steep ascents and descents that can result in more effort on the muscles in your legs. Running downhill can strengthen your muscles since it demands your muscles to stretch. Keep an eye out for running on trails can also carry danger of injury, especially in the event of falling or slips. Make sure you choose trails that are either downhill or uphill, with moderate slopes. If you are climbing, take short strides, and be sure to land in the middle of your foot to ensure greater stability. Also, you must create a routine. While descending, you should also reduce your steps. Be sure to wear appropriate footwear to ensure that you're able to hold on the ground.

* Water is often utilized as a means of rehab for people suffering from injuries to their calves or legs, aqua running can help improve the strength of muscles. This is due to greater resistance to water compared to the air (about 800 times). Due to this, it is necessary to work harder to get yourself pushing to the same length on water that you would on the land. Running in water that is lower than waist deep is likely to make the lower leg muscles to work harder.

Proper Breathing

Create a relaxed breathing routine that works for the pace you are running. It is important to breath deeply to facilitate the exchange of oxygen, which will improve the capacity of your lungs and increase endurance. For those who are just beginning, focus on breathing deeply and discover your technique that works for you. This will distract you whenever you are ready to give up. Inefficient breathing can result in side stitches. Side stitches cause a cramp that is felt throughout the lower part of the body. They're typically observed in people who are newbies. A deep breath can eliminate side stitches, even if you're just beginning.

Breathing through your mouth is an effective method because it allows you to take in the oxygen that you require and exhale air in large quantities too. The breath through your nose draws lower levels of oxygen. Breathing through the mouth assists in keeping the muscles of the face relaxed. breath through the nose makes jaw muscles tense and then tightens the neck muscles and shoulders. The mouth should be slightly opened for mouth breathing to ease.

The ability to breathe in tune with the beat is another method of efficient breathing while running. This can help regulate the rate of your breathing, and keeps your heart rate in check. Discover music that is aligned with your breathing rate and pace. Take an MP3 player with you or sing along to the beat of the song.

If none of these methods work If you are not satisfied, try this. The breathing rhythm is timed according to the steps. Make sure you are breathing in sync with your movements in a manner similar to 2:2. This means that you inhale by two steps and exhale with two steps. Try 3-3:

inhale for 3 steps before exhaling with three steps. Breathing at your own pace allows your body in matching it to the intensity of your workout.

Average Speed and Distance

What is the average jogging time and distance? The speed and distance depend on endurance. Average jogging speeds are between 4-5.5 miles per hour, but it depends on the level of fitness and the height of the person. Build and height affect the stride length and the speed. Running speed can be maintained through strong endurance and stamina.

If you've now discovered the reason why many people are considering jogging as beneficial and what the benefits are of jogging Are you confident that it is healthy for you? Set your goals. What do you hope to accomplish? Make them achievable and work towards achieving your goals.

Hal Higdon, author and writer has written a book for people who are looking to get started. The process is easy and you will only require 30 minutes over the course of 30 days. This doesn't have to be completed every single day. It could be adjusted to run every other day, or as often as 3-4 times per week, however you must it must be completed for a full 30 days.

• Walk out and take 15 minutes of walking in one direction, then turn around and return. This is the first day of your life and you have completed an hour of walking.

For a good start to your exercise start by walking for the first 10 minutes. It is not necessary to run or jog.

*To finish your workout, run for the final five minutes.

* In the last 15 minutes, you can run or jog at a moderate pace, but don't push your self.

* Here's what you'll do during the 15 minutes between in the middle 15 minutes: run for 30 seconds then walk for a recovery then jog for 30 secs then walk for a recovery repeating this process

After your body has become adjusted to the exercise, you can alternately jog and walk for 30 seconds at a time.

It is advised for healthy adults to exercise jogging and running for at least three times per week. Each session should last between 20 and 60 minutes. For aerobic exercises keep your cardiovascular rate for at minimum 20 minutes in order to reap the benefits.

Stamina is essential for enduring jogging. To build stamina, do interval training. Once you've warmed up you can jog at a steady pace for five minutes. Then intensify the pace and keep it up for one minute before going back to the speed you are comfortable with for 5 minutes. This is an active rehabilitation. If you are a beginner there is a different version for a start. Walk briskly as an active recuperation. This ratio for active and work is 1:5. You can alter this ratio if you feel it does not suit you or is too heavy for your needs. The work is increased gradually each week by 30 seconds as well as reducing your the active recuperation by 30 seconds. In the wake of this first instance next week, it will be the 1.5:4.5 ratio.

The main purpose behind these programs is to begin slow, then, pay attention to your body. If you hurry, you're susceptible to injury.

Best Time

The best time to run?

It was discovered that body temperatures dip at the beginning of the day and rises to its maximum in the later afternoon. A few athletes can perform very well when they have the body temperature being high.

The health of your body may not be performing at its peak during the early morning hours. Body temperatures are poor, muscles are rigid, the lung's function has been diminished, and energy levels are lower. In this state the body is working hard to get fit and increase the risk of an injury. A few athletes see this as a mental exercise and the greater effort they exert, the better they experience. Boxers work out and practice their running in the mornings.

However there are many aspects to take into consideration. Each body's clock is individual. It is also determined by family and work or other obligations. A few people jog early at dawn due to less pollution and traffic in the morning, before going to work. Some discover that if they run at the beginning of the day and sleep more soundly later in the night. The study found that running early in the morning before breakfast, helps to lose weight more quickly because it burns more fat for energy instead of carbs. Even the night-owls don't subscribe with this and prefer hitting the sleep button.

There are others who manage to run during lunch breaks due to obligations in the morning, and throughout the day.

A few people enjoy jogging during the afternoon to ease the pressure caused by their work, or simply because that is the time they can be available.

A few prefer running at night. Some people don't want to do it due to security concerns, but certain people are keeping away from the harsh rays of sun. Exercise relieves stress. anxiety is the majority of times caused by the pressures of working, which is why many people prefer to jog at night.

Many people would prefer to exercise at night due to similar reasons to the ones discussed. They would like to stay away from the scorching heat. The traffic is lower and there's less pollution. There is a belief that people can sleep better after an exhausting exercise in the evening.

It's just that there's insufficient evidence to determine which timing is the best.

A professional suggested workout for a few weeks at various timings of the day: early morning, lunch afternoon, evening, and even in the evening. After that, evaluate the results. What we know for sure being able to change to whatever. If we can train our body to exercise at a specific interval, the body will be taught how to handle it, adjust to it and eventually become successful. If you are outdoors, don't neglect to take into account the weather conditions too.

Chapter 13: Jogging Injuries And Treatment

The majority of injuries sustained by joggers can be avoided and prevented. Based on the Dr. Matthew Matava of the American Orthopaedic Society for Sports Medicine the most frequent cause of injuries is a lack of training due to a insufficient stretching, rapid shifts in speed, hill-training as well as interval training and the inability to rest between workouts.

Be aware of the risk of injury. Be aware of the different kinds of pain that can occur caused by injuries. You should be able to distinguish between emergency or not. Be aware of the risks that come with running and learn how to avoid them.

Acute Injuries

Soreness that develops after a delayed onset (DOMS) is among the most frequently and most debated subject in the field of running or jogging. The issue is DOMS. If exercise is too strenuous for our bodies, and there's not sufficient oxygen available to produce energy, the body searches for alternatives to energy sources and turns to producing it via anaerobically. This means, with no oxygen. The triphosphate adenosine (ATP) is a energy molecule that is used by muscles for fuel. By glycolysis, glucose can be converted into the pyruvate. When oxygen is present, pyruvate is subjected to aerobic metabolism in which ATP is the result. When oxygen levels are low the body transforms the pyruvate to lactate, which allows sugar breakdown to allow ATP production to go on. If the process is not stopped the build-up of lactate occurs in muscles, causing an increase in muscle acidity, and disrupting various metabolisms. This is part of our body's defense system that prevents damage for life and helps conserve energy. After the body has recovered and oxygen levels are increased and aerobic metabolism can be again facilitated. The accumulation of lactic acid within the muscles can be the cause discomfort and burning sensations when exercising. The lactic acid gets flushed out of the body in less than an hour. The pain is prevented by drinking enough fluids before, throughout, and following jogging. If you're in the beginning stage, don't let the pain rule over your fitness and goals, work out often because when you exercise regularly, you will have lesser glucose available to burn and consequently, there'll be lesser acid build-up. When you jog and your body begins to "feel the burn" shift to a recovery stage however, don't stop because your body is saying that you're exaggerating, therefore allow your body minutes to recuperate. Others recommend keeping track of your the rate of heartbeat during exercise for determining your threshold of anaerobic exercise. While speed may not be the indicator that you're putting excessive effort. Instead, pay attention to your body's signalling. Once you are at home, follow this rule: PRICE (protect against injury, rest or ice compression and elevating). If the pain persists take a break and take a break.

Delayed-onset soreness (DOMS) is an extreme form of muscle soreness that is associated with a loss of range of movement and strength. It usually occurs between 24-72 hours post-exercise. The reason for this is that the muscles are stretched but are not used to it, causing the muscles to become damaged and then sore. The pain could be described as an aching, dull pain that causes stiffness as well as pain to the point of contact. The affected muscle displays inflammation and tenderness. It is able to heal up to 7 days post-exercise. When you have DOMS, although the muscles might be aching it is still able to be completed even though it might result in pain during the first few minutes of the workout. When you are subjected to the same exercises, the injured muscles adapt and recovers rapid. A gradual increase in intensity may help prevent DOMS. Resolve the DOMS issue by keeping the exercise routine. If you are experiencing persistent pain The massage and hot baths or a sauna could assist.

The delayed-onset soreness of muscles (DOMS) can be described as a type I strain. The most basic definition of strain would be injury to the tendon or muscle The term strain can be described as pulled muscles. Muscles are connected to joints via tendon. It can manifest as and stiffness. It can also cause swelling and a decreased functioning. The muscle may also be bruised when it is common. Apply the PRICE principle as the initial treatment for muscle strains.

*P -- Guard against further injuries

* R -Limit activity, sleep

* I -I - Ice therapy

* C - Compression

* E Increase the entire area

Ice therapy helps reduce swelling and pain, while compression is also a similar result. Place ice on the injury location for 15 minutes every three or four times during the daily.

Sprains can cause injuries to the ligament. Ligaments are fibrous tissues which connect bones to one another. Sprains can be classified according to intensity, extent of tears in tissues, pain swelling and state of joint.

The first degree of sprain is characterized by a little tear as well as swelling and pain and the body is functioning normally and power.

The second degree strain is evident when there is a significant degree of pain, tear and swelling. It also occurs in cases where strength and function is impaired.

The third degree strain is the worst due to the complete rupture of the ligament. There is significant swelling and pain as well as diminished strength and functionality.

Take note of your injury. If you are unable running or jog immediately stop. If you notice a deformity and you feel severe swelling and pain, you must place the injured area on ice and contact a medical professional. If there is something that is straining, adhere to the PRICE rule.

First aid principles helps reduce swelling, and aid to speed up healing. The pads and splints secure and protect the region. The recommended rest period is during the following 24 to 72 hours so that the healing process can begin. It is recommended to apply ice for 15 to 20 minutes, three or four every day. Do not directly apply the ice and cover it up with a towel, or put it in an frozen bag. An elastic bandage is ideal for applying compression and providing support however, do not make the bandage too tightly, as you don't want to limit the blood flow. It is possible to maintain compression while you sleep. The injured region should be elevated to reduce swelling. If the injury is not severe begin gentle exercise around the area affected one to three days after the injury. If you're unable to lift weights and/or your symptoms become worse over the following 24 hours, you should seek out professional medical attention.

Metatarsalgia causes inflammation to the sole of the foot as a result of the pressure that is placed on it. It can also result from an abnormality in the structure of the foot as well as inappropriate footwear. Treatment options include ice therapy orthotics and footwear that has an arch support, or insoles to are able to absorb the impact. Softer running surfaces will help reduce pressure on the area affected.

Shin splints, also more commonly referred to as medial tibial stress syndrome is an irritation of muscles and the tendons. The symptoms include discomfort in the lower leg. Keep in mind that exercises with high-impact could cause shin splints to develop, similarly, active rests. Active rest is when you do low-impact workouts. One suggested workout is aqua jogging, with feet that are not at the floor of the water. The first step is to treat the injury with ice and then rest. The amount of resting required for the affected limb will be contingent on how severe the injury. Avoid shin splints by gradually intensifying your exercises to not more than 10% each week. Switch to a smoother surface. Orthotics can also be utilized to avoid repeat incidence. If not treated this can cause stress fractures.

Meniscal tear is the most common injury that affects the knee and can be caused by a abrupt twisting or turning the knee. Meniscus is the cartilage that surrounds the knee. A meniscal tear can be identified by a swelling, pain and locking of the joint, and the knee buckling. A small tear may present with slight discomfort and swelling and heals within two to three weeks. The moderate tear is characterized by painfulness on either middle or side of the knee. Swelling grows in two to three days. The knee is stiff and the ability to bend is restricted. The symptoms can last from 1 to two weeks, but they can quickly recur when the knee becomes bent or is over-used. In the case of severe tears that cause knee pain, the knee will buckle and will feel as though it's about to be able to give way. A joint locking issue may occur as an area of the damaged ligament becomes in the way in straightening the knee. Treatment for this condition is with physical therapy. Based on the extent of tear, surgeries can be performed can be performed to fix or remove the cartilage tear. Preventing the tear involves wearing proper shoes, stretching, and strengthening exercises for the hamstrings calves, quadriceps and. Muscles that are strong can assist in absorbing the strain.

A different acute ache which is not common but should be considered is chest pain. It is taken carefully because it's usually connected to the heart and important organs located within the chest cavity. Many joggers and long-time runners have complained about chest pain when exercising and running, but they don't know how to deal with it. The chest pain experienced by runners could result from inefficient breathing or a tired pectoral muscle.

Additional research on the subject has revealed the following. The precordial catch syndrome (PCS) which is sometimes referred to as The Texidor's Twinge is a form of chest pain commonly experienced by infants and adults. PCS is characterized by acute, painful pain generally on the left of the chest. It gets worse when breathing and moving. Due to this typical chest pain, many children as well as young adults believe they're suffering from an attack on their heart. It can last anywhere from two to three seconds or just a couple of minutes. In very rare instances, it could extend to thirty minutes. There's no evidence on the frequency and incidence however, the majority of times, it is gone in a short time. There's no cure for PCS. Once the pain has gone away the jogger will be left with worry and fear in the event that chest pain could signal a heart attack.

Angina pectoris is a different kind of chest pain that is caused by the lack of oxygen supply to the heart's muscles and could be related to the lack of blood flow to the blood vessels within the heart. The chest pain can be a tight, heavy feeling and burning. It can also be described as squeezing or even choking. It can occur in various parts of the body, such as the back, epigastrium jaw, neck as well as shoulders. It may be associated with excessive sweating and breathing difficulties. Angina is often due to physical or emotional tension. It can be worse when you have the stomach full and also in frigid temperatures. If you experience this, contact your physician immediately. Angina may mean a variety of kinds of things, but it all points at the heart.

One of the main causes of chest pain is a heart attack. Heart attacks are because of a cut or severing in the supply of blood to coronary arteries, also known as the arteries that supply blood to the heart. The cholesterol and fat build up in arteries and create the formation of a plaque. If this plaque is broken and platelets accumulate at the location and block blood flow. If blood flow to heart muscle is cut off it leads to the death of muscles, which causes permanent injury to the heart. It is said that chest pains can feel tight, squeezey, and painful. It can radiate into the jaw, arms the neck, back, and the epigastrium. A shortness of breath, nausea and sweaty palms are also possible. If pain doesn't ease within five minutes, you should call to get emergency medical assistance. The earlier detection improves the chances of the survival.

The risk of dehydration is high during running or jogging, that is the reason why everyone is constantly reminded to drink water. When you are in a high-intensity physical environment it is common for the body to lose water. can be lost due to sweat breath, heat, and breathing. The first signs of dehydration are thirst and the mouth becoming dry, nausea, and decreased urinary flow, mild signs like extreme thirst, dizziness, weak and severe signs like cramps as well as chills and disorientation. To fight the symptoms of dehydration drink two glasses of water for 1 an hour prior to running/jogging. Drink one glass of water every 15 minutes during your exercise, and then take a drink immediately after. The stomach is able to absorb approximately 1 glass of fluid per

15 minutes. This means it can't take in more at once. It is possible to consume beverages for sports, which is also a good source of electrolytes. When you exercise and your the amount of urine you drink is less or more concentrated which means you're dehydrated and should drink more. If you weigh yourself prior to and following running or jogging, you'll weigh the same if you are you are properly hydrated.

Intoxication from water, on the contrary, occurs due to drinking excessive amounts of drinking water in a short amount of duration. Distance runners tend to this, in order to stop loss of water. When a significant quantity of water is consumed within a brief duration, it can cause the condition known as hyponatremia. It is a reduction in blood levels of sodium which is an indication of imbalance in electrolytes. The sodium helps with the exchange of fluids as well as electrolytes that are not in the cells of the body. It also plays a role to regulating blood pressure. Intoxication by water can cause nausea and vomiting as well as confusion and headaches, weakness of the muscles as well as seizures. Coma or death could be a outcome if intoxication is serious. Remember the consequences of drinking water, but consider water as your best partner. Water is involved in many aspects of the body's function. It prevents cramps and muscle tension regulates body temperature, helps prevent constipation, flushes out the skin of toxins, and maintains its moisture and firmness.

One of the most common issues when running is the possibility of fainting. Syncope, or fainting, is defined in The Merck Manual as "a sudden, brief loss of consciousness". The functioning of the brain is impaired. It can occur during exercise because there isn't enough blood flow is provided by the heart to deliver oxygen required by the body. This is known as exertion or syncope. The same can occur when exercising, because as the blood pressure decreases as does blood flow. The volume drops, however the muscles' blood vessels remain dilation. When this happens, the arterioles dilate in order to provide oxygen for the muscles, and veins are expanded to help transport metabolic substances that are discarded. If the amount of blood is reduced, however the blood vessels in the distal part are filled with blood, it decreases the pressure and leads to a faint. Doctor. Christopher Bell of Intermountain Healthcare says that to avoid fainting, "...`hot volunteers or walkers' staff take finishers' names and continue walking them when they cross the the line. When you walk on following your finish, you continue working those muscles in your legs to pump blood until your heart system is able to recover from the exertion." The point is the perfect opportunity to demonstrate that cool-downs are crucial.

Hypothermia is a different risk that when you exercise outdoors. Outside, there's no means to measure the temperature of your body. You'll need to trust your gut instincts about the way you feel. There are many variables that can lead to hypothermia.

* Air temperature

* Clothing that is wet. It's not the only thing you'll be able to achieve when wearing sweaty clothing. If you're wearing a winter coat on the outside, but your inside clothing is soiled with sweat then you'll start losing heat. If you're not certain about the temperature, pack more clothes and wear jackets that allow you to adjust layers using zippers.

* Wind. Wind won't aid to keep you warm, especially in the case of sweat. Evaporative cooling occurs when the wind strikes your body. Even if you aren't feeling windy the movement of air while you run aids in cooling by evaporation.

* Rain. Make sure you check the weather predictions before running because being in the rain won't help your cause.

* Exhaustion. When you are fatigued, no body heat is created to keep you warm.

* Night and evening. Running when the sun is in the sky will give you heat from the outside while jogging when the sun isn't up will helps to lower the temperature.

The signs of hypothermia are sensations of feeling cold, tired, or have muscular tension and chills, which is mild hypothermia. Be aware of warning symptoms of hypothermia moderate, that include slurred speech lack of coordination and pale lips. Also, you may notice blue fingers and eardrums. The signs of severe hypothermia are shaking at a rapid pace, talking exhausted, drowsiness, or exhaustion. To prevent hypothermia in particular during winter, you should wear at minimum three layers of clothing. Wear thermal clothing, as it aids in the generation and retention of the heat. Wearing cotton clothes that do won't help you stay comfortable because it stores sweat. In the middle layer, wear clothing that is made from wool or synthetic fibers that will help you stay cozy. Your outer layer should comprise an waterproof jacket with a zips, certain jackets come with several layers. You can adjust the temperature using the zipper. Keep your head covered to retain the body temperature and don't forget to put on gloves. The overdressing of your head will limit your movements. Recognize the first signs of hypothermia. Get warm immediately.

Another thing to consider. The process of exhaustion causes heat and your body's ability to manage the temperature. Similar to hypothermia it is potentially life-threatening. The chance of suffering from heat exhaustion increases with temperatures that are hot. The signs of exhaustion include great bumps, fatigue nausea, headache, dizziness and vomiting. Also, it can cause a the skin is clammy and cool. Before going out for a run, make sure you look up the weather forecast. high humidity and heat can affect the body. If you are in the midst of extreme heat warnings you should stay in the shade. Keep yourself hydrated and follow it up with walks. Drink water prior to jogging or run, as well as following. The drinks you drink during and after your workout will to replenish electrolytes as well. A splash of water can aid in cooling down via Evaporative cooling. A heat stroke is an medical emergency. If you're alone and you feel the first symptoms of exhaustion due to heat, you should relax at a cooler location. take off your clothes to aid in helping your body cool down as well as ice packs for the lower back, the groin, and neck can help ease the heat. In the summer, jog during the hour of the morning when temperatures are at their lowest. Choose to run close to the bodies of water such as oceans, lakes, rivers where temperatures are lower and a breeze helps to disperse the heat. Dress in light colors as they reflect the UV rays of the sun. Clothing that is dark is absorbed by heat and makes the body's temperature increase. Use a visor.

Humidity is another factor to think about. When humidity is higher which means that the amount of moisture in the air is greater and you'll feel more hot as sweat does not evaporate in the air. Always be sure to verify the weather forecast prior to running. Hydrate. If the humidity is very high, you do not want to slide to the point of exhaustion. It is a good rule of thumb that if the humidity exceeds 40%, you are hydrated. One other thing to consider is your humidity index. This is the result of humidity and temperature that gives you an idea of how is the actual feeling out there.

Everyone handles temperatures and humidity differently. it could be due to the process of acclimatization. Additionally, there are other variables. Size of the body influences how you manage heat. With larger body weight will be more insulated, and the temperatures are high meaning that the body is able to generate much more heat and is susceptible to being overheated. Another reason is age. with age the sweat glands lose their capacity to make sweat. Consequently your body's capability to cool itself.

A different risk is hypoglycemia. No matter if you're suffering from type 1 or 2 diabetes, or hypoglycemia reactive, you should not allow it to hinder your exercising. In hypoglycemia, the blood sugars is not as high. But before you start, seek medical advice first. The doctor will evaluate your medical condition before determining if you're clear, begin walking. It's essential to be aware of the relationship between eating and exercising. The foods that have low glycemic Index are preferred because they take more slowly. Monitoring the levels of your blood sugar require continuous monitoring of your blood sugar levels. The signs of hypoglycemia include the appearance of cold sweats as well as double vision, hungry and headache. It is advised to eat a meal 1 hour before exercising and eat small portions of food regularly. If you are experiencing signs of hypoglycemia, you should take an insulin tablet. If you are having difficulty controlling the sugar levels of your body through exercises, speak to your doctor or a dietician. Make sure you wear comfortable shoes. You do not want blisters.

Overuse Injury

Plantar fasciitis refers to the inflammation of connective tissue on the heel often referred to by the name of "policeman's heel". The connective tissue affected in the plantar fascia begins at the heel and extends all the way to the toes. The inflammation of this type is due to long-term carrying weight. When you jog, your feet take on the load and because of the intense impact exercise, feet are able to absorb up to three times the body weight.

It is not just weight that can be a element to the accident. It is said that pain is experienced in the heel area, mild, and noticeable within the first couple of steps during the day. Also, there is difficulty stretching the foot to bring it toward the side of the. Treatment options include relaxation, massage, stretching and physical therapy. It also includes heating and cold therapy as well as orthotics and anti-inflammatory medication. Massage therapy can bring relief immediately. The stretching of the Achilles tendon as well as the plantar fascia before going to bed can reduce pain during the initial stages of your day. Another method of relieving pain is using the ice treatment and mixing the application of heating therapy. Orthotics that are custom-made can help ease the pain. Good support shoes as well as a good cushioning can ease the pain as well.

A foot stress fracture results from the stress or fatigue that comes from regular exercise caused by the weight of. The leg is a target for stress fractures. could be the result of a hairline or complete fracture in the fibula or tibia. The symptoms include painful and tenderness around the fractured bone. The discomfort is intense in the beginning of an exercise, but it becomes milder during the middle part of the workout, but it will become severe at the conclusion. The appearance of bruising could be. It is important to rest and stay immobile in order for the bone affected to heal. You can also include Vitamin D and calcium supplements in the diet. Running can be resumed slowly in the course of one to two months. To avoid recurrence, run on surfaces that are soft and then change your running shoes once you have used them for 400 to 500 miles.

Exertional compartment syndrome occurs when exercise is involved and can be defined as a reduction in the supply of blood to a leg or limb affected. It's characterised by tightness or swelling. It can also cause impairment of the limb affected. It is a serious injury that requires prompt medical care. Surgery is typically the first choice for treatment.

Achilles tendonitis occurs due to excessive use of the Achilles tendon. It manifests as discomfort and tightness within the calf muscles, which is typically due to the hill-running. It takes time for the injury to heal due to no enough activity of cells or blood flow in the tendon of Achilles. Treatments can include stretching, rest Ice therapy, anti-inflammatory drugs in combination with elastic compression and heels pads. Heel pads reduce tension over the tendon. The application of an elastic compression bandages can help lessen stiffness during the day make sure that the pressure is gentle to medium in order not to restrict blood flow. It is likewise recommended to consult a professional for help as it could cause Achilles tendon rupture. Anti-inflammatory drugs that are non-steroidal can reduce pain and swelling. The cause of this can be avoided by exercise to strengthen the calves.

Pain in the Patellofemoral Joint is caused by distance running, changing conditions, as well as changes in footwear. It manifests as a pain in the kneecap. Treatment options include ice and cutting down on knee activities until discomfort is relieved. Then look at non-impact activities such as running or swimming. Perform quadriceps exercises to keep the kneecap in place. Wearing shoes that have good arch support, or orthotics that are custom made could help lessen the burden on knees.

Patellar tendonitis, also called "jumper's knee" presents as the sensation of pain that is accompanied by aches and at first, the patellar tendon increases in size and can cause tears to the tendon. It is divided into 4 phases:

* Stage 1 pain is evident immediately following the exercise, and there is no impairment of the functional.

* Stage 2 pain is evident both during and following the exercise without functional impairment.

The pain in Stage 3 is exacerbated in the course of and after an activity as well as functional impairment

In Stage 4, there is a an entire tear in the tendon. Surgery is required to be carried out

If surgery isn't necessary take a break from the knee until it is pain-free, then use ice treatment, and non-steroidal antiinflammatory medicines will help reduce swelling and pain.

The cause of bursitis is inflammation of the bursa the tiny sacs of liquid which cushion joints and provide lubrication. Prepatellar knee arthritis, also called "housemaid's knee" is the irritation of the preatellar bursa located between the kneecap and skin. In the case of joggers, it can be caused by putting a lot of stress on the kneecap. The phrase "housemaid's Knee" originated from the days where housekeepers cleaned floors with their knees. The condition is characterised by tenderness, pain, swelling, and redness over the kneecap. It can be due to trauma or repetitive use or rheumatoid arthritis. It also results caused by uric acid deposits. It can also be caused by infection and manifest as symptoms of fever. In addition, knee pain can increase and can result in stiffness which means that the flexibility of the knee becomes restricted. Relieve, ice therapy and anti-inflammatory medicines are all typical treatment options. Based on the assessment of the physician, the fluid must be removed and the affected bursa treated by cortisone. In the event of infection and antibiotic treatment is recommended, it's the treatment option and in the event of need, aspiration or the removal of the affected bursa could be necessary. Another kind of knee pain is known as infrapatellar joint bursitis. It's is also known by the name of "jumper's knee", the bursa that lies below the kneecap has become damaged and can cause a jump injury. Another type of knee bursitis, also known as anserine bursitis. The bursa affected is the one located in the inside of your knee. It is more common among the overweight and is felt on both hills and up. The treatment for infrapatellar and anserine bursitis includes rest, treatment with ice, an anti-inflammatory pain medication.

The hip bursa is another place that is prone to inflammation. The condition is known as trochanteric bursitis. It causes an inflammation of the bursa which lies on the outside of the hip. Ischial bursitis causes inflammation of the bursa, which is located in the upper buttock region. The two injuries are characterized by an uncomfortable, constant pain that increases as you walk uphill. The pain that is felt on the ischial musculature can be is a result of sitting for long periods on hard surfaces. It is sometimes referred to for its slang name "weaver's bottom" or "tailor's bottom." Itchyness is often present while lying on the area affected. Most treatment options include treatment with ice, rest as well as anti-inflammatory pain and inflammation medicines. Also, it is recommended to lower weight in order to lessen load on the area affected. The stretching exercises can increase your the strength of muscles and reduce the load. It is recommended to wear appropriate footwear to reduce the load. If the condition isn't yet been solved, it's crucial to steer clear of stress, running on hills as well as using the staircase. If there is an infection it is followed by fever. This requires treatment with antibiotics and perhaps drainage. Get help from a professional.

Iliotibial band syndrome (ITBS) is a common knee injury for runners. Iliotibial band refers to fascia's band connects to the exterior of the knee. It extends from the outside of the thigh. It then runs through the patella's inside and wraps around the tibia. It helps keep the knee from moving during all times of activity. The reason for inflammation is repeated knee movements, and when your knee bends,, it results in tension on the ligament as it rubs on the lateral epicondyle of the femoral scapula, that can be described as the bony prominence on the femur located on the left part of the knee as well as when the knee is extended, the knee gets strained again. The injury manifests as painful, sharp pain that stings at the outside of the knee throughout the exercise and will get worse as you move. It also causes thickening of the ligament. Any high-impact activity has to be resisted. A combination of several elements is the reason for this, and they include fitness habits, biomechanics and imbalances in muscles. When you are in the acute stage you should opt for minimal or no impacts aerobic activities like aqua jogging. It relieves tension and strain off of the muscle. Ice therapy is recommended since it can reduce swelling and improves circulation to the region. Pain and anti-inflammatory medications may assist. If you are sleeping, make sure to place an extra pillow between the knees in order to reduce the pressure around the band. Once the discomfort and inflammation is gone, massages can be administered. Contact a physical therapist or massage therapy. A foam roller is a great way to ease tight muscles. Stretches can help to lengthen the band. ITBS is preventable by switching out your running shoes at least every 400 to 500 miles. It is thought to occur each three or four months, dependent on the amount and regularity of jogging. At this point, it is apparent that shoes lose around half their shock absorption capabilities. Increase the distance, or add an gradual incline in your workout and be sure to stay clear of the uneven surface. Always do a regular warm-up or cool downs.

Sciatica is a condition that causes compression on the sciatic nerve. The symptoms include pain in the back of the lower torso or buttocks or buttocks, but can also manifest with numbness or weakness, or a sensation of tingling on the foot or leg. Sciatica typically is result of herniated discs. that impinge onto the sciatic nerve. The other causes are tumors, injuries, slip discs or disc bulge and muscles spasms. The fact that you jog does not cause sciatica isn't the reason however, the discomfort can slow your progress and the force of impact could cause tension in the current nerve compression. The treatment includes resting in bed to relieve pressure on this nerve. Weight loss and heating packs. The body's mechanics must be correct. Exercise can help to strengthen your back.

Chapter 14: Safety Jogging Tips

Once you've mastered how to jog take time for your exercise routine. These are some tips may be helpful to you.

* Eat a healthy diet. Fast food and fad diets will hinder your progress. While you're required to the energy for your exercise, however, avoid fueling it with processed foods, fat-laden food or sweet foods. Make sure you are consuming nutritious and fresh foods.

Remember to drink plenty of water prior to starting. Take note of any indicators of loss of hydration. The waist packs are available on the marketplace, and they is a great way to hold water so that you are hydrated whenever you want to.

www.ingramcontent.com/pod-product-compliance
Lightning Source LLC
Chambersburg PA
CBHW051726020426
42333CB00014B/1182